MODELS FOR NURSING 2

Edited by

JANE SALVAGE MSc BA RGN
Director, Nursing Developments
King's Fund Centre for Health Services Development
London

and

BETTY KERSHAW MSc SRN RNT
Director of Nursing Education
Stockport and
Tameside & Glossop Health Authorities

With 11 contributors

SCUTARI PRESS
London

KU-475-047

√c

| MEDICAL LIBRARY |
| QUEEN'S MEDICAL CENTRE |

Class   WY 86 MOD
Fund   JAN 20
Book
No.   6200478762

© Scutari Press 1990

A division of Scutari Projects, the publishing company of the Royal College of Nursing.

All rights reserved. No part of this publication may be reproduced, stored in a retrieval system or transmitted, in any form or by any means, electronic, mechanical, photocopying or other-wise, without the prior permission of Scutari Press, Viking House, 17–19 Peterborough Road, Harrow, Middlesex, HA1 2AX, England.

First published 1990

British Library Cataloguing in Publication Data

Models for nursing.
  2.
  I. Kershaw, Betty II. Salvage, Jane
  1. Medicine. Nursing
  610.73

  ISBN 1-871364-26-4

Typeset by Blackpool Typesetting Services Limited
Printed and bound in Great Britain by Biddles Ltd, Guildford

Contributors

DIANA CARTER BA MSc RGN SCM DipN RNT is lecturer in nursing studies at the University of Glasgow.

HELEN CHALMERS BA RGN RNT DipN is senior tutor, Continuing Education Department, Bath Health Authority.

PAUL CHAPMAN RMN RNT DipN CertEd is professional officer with the Confederation of Health Service Employees.

CHRIS ELLIOTT-CANNON RNMH RNT CertEd is senior tutor (mental handicap), Stockport Health Authority.

ALAN GLASPER BA RSCN RGN NDN CertEd RNT is head of department and lecturer in nursing studies in the Faculty of Medicine and Nursing Studies, University of Southampton.

CHRISTINE HENDERSON MA SRN SCM DipN MTD is head of midwifery and related studies, Birmingham and Solihull College of Midwifery.

ANNE JONES RGN NDN is a district nursing sister with South Bedfordshire Health Authority.

BETTY KERSHAW MSc SRN RNT is director of nursing education, Stockport and Tameside & Glossop Health Authorities.

JANE SALVAGE MSc BA RGN is director, nursing developments, at the King's Fund Centre for Health Services Development.

PAM SMITH PhD MSc BNurs RNT is senior nurse, research, in Bloomsbury Health Authority.

BARBARA VAUGHAN MSc SRN DipN RCNT RNT DANS is senior lecturer, School of Nursing Studies, University of Wales College of Medicine.

MIKE WALSH BA RGN PGCE DipN is senior lecturer in nursing at Bristol Polytechnic.

STEVE WRIGHT MSc RGN RCNT RNT DipN DANS is consultant nurse, care of the elderly, Tameside Nursing Development Unit, Tameside and Glossop Health Authority.

Contents

Preface

Since the first volume of *Models for Nursing* was published in 1986, it has become increasingly apparent that nurses are developing model-based care in all areas of practice. Many nurses are evaluating these innovations and are introducing them alongside other valued initiatives such as family-centred care, primary nursing and the movement of long-stay patients into the community. Others are incorporating health or patient education programmes into model-based care. As usual, the innovative nurse, midwife and health visitor is moving care ahead on more than one front.

This approach makes even more sense in the light of the constraints facing nurses as they strive to deliver the high quality of care our clients deserve. Any approach to nursing that aids staff retention and job satisfaction and improves individualised patient care must be welcome to staff, patients, managers and teachers alike.

This volume, like the previous one, aims to help all nurses, whether students or qualified staff, who are considering changing practice or using new ideas in care. It offers them the opportunity to explore for themselves initiatives taken by colleagues working in similar fields under the same constraints; learning from peers is one of the most valuable forms of education.

This book is not meant to act as a vehicle for new model exposition. Rather it is a text that describes how nurses in a wide range of settings have developed model-based practice to suit their own particular environment. As such it should prove useful to students on statutory as well as degree courses. Qualified staff should also find something of relevance to their own practice; teachers and managers may also benefit from the examples offered. In short, the book will help all nurses understand how the texts of the theorists have been translated into practice.

Like the previous volume, this book augments the work of Aggleton and Chalmers, Wright, Pearson and Vaughan, Walsh, Collister and others who explored model-based practice in a wide variety of settings. Many of the authors in this book, however, are publishing their experiences for the first time, bringing new ideas to professional scrutiny. The chapters on model-based care in midwifery and mental handicap are especially welcome as examples of other fields in which the ideas are being explored.

The terms 'she' to describe the nurse and 'he' to refer to the patient are used only for clarity when alternatives are unavoidable, and do not endorse a sexist approach.

We would like to thank all our contributors, especially those writing for the first time. We would also like to acknowledge the help received from Barbara Vaughan and Steve Wright, who have discussed the original ideas with us and encouraged us along the way. We must also place on record our appreciation of our publisher, Patrick West, for his patient nurturing of both volumes.

Change in nursing practice is now constant, inevitable and well established. It offers nurses ever-present challenges. We hope this book will, in a small way, help them meet those challenges in a creative and open spirit.

BETTY KERSHAW
JANE SALVAGE
June 1989

Models for Nursing 2
Edited by B Kershaw and J Salvage
© 1990 Scutari Press

1

Introduction

JANE SALVAGE

In 1985, when Betty Kershaw and I compiled our first collection of papers on nursing models (Kershaw & Salvage 1986), the subject was something of a novelty in British nursing. We had been involved in mounting the first models conference in the UK, and we noted then that the interest in relating theories and models to clinical practice was accelerating. That trend has continued in the intervening years, to the extent that the question many practitioners are asked today is not 'Are you using a nursing model?', but 'Which model are you using?'

This explosion of interest is in many ways welcome to those nurses who believe that an exploration of the issues that models raise is healthy, relevant and appropriate to contemporary practice. Nevertheless, the implication of asking the question 'Which model?' – as though the need to work within a specific theoretical perspective is already taken for granted – highlights the dangers of embracing new and in many respects untested ideas without due caution. Nurses should not be made to feel guilty if their practice is not based on an explicit model, nor should it be assumed that all progressive practitioners are using one. Many other approaches to nursing practice can be justified as equally beneficial to patients and clients.

Nearly every contributor to this collection is alert to these dangers, and many cite the introduction of the nursing process as an alarming precedent. This too was a novelty, though partly based on existing practice. It too came winging across the Atlantic Ocean and was seized on as the solution to all our problems. It was often forced on unwilling or uncomprehending staff by over-enthusiastic managers who failed to appreciate that change would take root only if it was 'owned' by practitioners themselves. Many senior nurses did not understand the full implications of the changes, while others ducked their responsibilities. The nursing process, like nursing models, was seen as inherently progressive although research and evaluation of its effects on patient care were only just beginning. The net result was that many ordinary nurses were alienated from a new approach which in fact had a great deal to offer.

Sadly, many nurses did not learn the lessons of the nursing process experience, and some of those mistakes are now being repeated with the spread of interest in nursing models. Similar stories are told of senior nurses or National Board officers who insist on model X being introduced by a certain date regardless of the views of practitioners. Many of these tales are probably apocryphal, but their very existence fuels the fears of nurses who are resistant to change. Although it is a mistake to equate the content of the innovation with the manner of its implementation, the stories reinforce the tendency to throw out the baby with the bathwater.

One major development since the publication of our first volume has been the growth of interest in primary nursing. If anything this has been seized on with even more alacrity as the answer to every nurse's prayer, to the extent that nursing models are virtually 'old hat'. If it has achieved nothing else, the enthusiasm for primary nursing has probably done nursing models a service by deflecting some of the heat! Yet the very same mistakes are being repeated with primary nursing, incurring the same risk of a backlash, which might discredit the ideas themselves rather than the way they are translated into practice.

Analysis of this rapid cycle of absorption of and reaction against new ideas could provide fascinating insights into modern nursing. What is it that nurses are seeking when they take up innovations and then drop them with such speed? What are the roots of this insatiable hunger for novelty? An understanding of this phenomenon would have to be based on examining modern nursing practice within its historical, political, social and economic context. The relationship between the quest for professional status and autonomy among influential sectors of the occupation, and the forced march towards fundamental change in the National Health Service, could provide the beginnings of a hypothesis.

The contributors to this volume cannot, however, be accused of merely jumping on bandwagons: none of them would claim that nursing models are a panacea. Yet they do not believe that models are valueless because they are sometimes introduced to practice in a clumsy, thoughtless or authoritarian way. All our contributors developed their ideas while based in clinical practice or working closely with practitioners in an educative role. Their views are based on clinical experience, and not purely on study and academic speculation, important as those activities are in developing nursing knowledge.

In all this debate, the need to identify and secure the support required for developing model-based nursing has become increasingly apparent. Many nurses who are enthused by the ideas nevertheless say that they cannot test them in practice because they do not have enough time, or money, or understanding managers, or forward-thinking staff. In this area, as in so many others, there is a dawning realisation of the need to explore not only the context of new ideas, but also the constraints on putting them into practice.

The current turmoil in the NHS – chronic funding problems exacerbated by the threat of wholesale but untested reform – is making nurses acutely aware of the context in which they carry out their work and the factors that prevent them from doing it as they would like to do it. At such a time it is understandable that many people feel less than enthusiastic about change; the changes already being forced upon them are more than enough to cope with, and introducing model-based practice is seen as no exception.

Exploring some of the issues surrounding the introduction of model-based nursing essentially means exploring the introduction of change of any kind. Here we are concerned particularly with models, but the issues are equally relevant to the nursing process, primary nursing or any other innovation. The task of facilitating or supporting a new development is often seen to be primarily one for the manager, but in a sense every nurse is a manager of the care she gives, so the issues are equally relevant to practitioners.

It may be a cliché to observe that change is a part of all our lives, but it is surprising what a difficult business we find it. There seems to be an innate human tendency to cling to familiarity, however stale or profitless or even painful it may be. Yet we must now come to terms with living in a world that is changing more rapidly than it has at any time in the history of human kind. The NHS reflects this state of flux: think of the plethora of changes it has recently undergone – reorganisations, major policy shifts, financial cuts, the attempted imposition of new marketplace values, to name only a few. Instead of regarding change as an unwelcome interference with our daily routine, we must start to view it as a way of life; to see it as a challenge rather than a threat. If nurses cannot learn to handle it creatively, they themselves will be the victims – as well as their patients.

Even if we learn to revalue change as a way of life, we must still acknowledge that it is usually painful, unfair, messy and long drawn out. However well intentioned it is, somebody somewhere will inevitably suffer, while even the proposed beneficiaries may undergo some painful ups and downs. It is all the more important, then, that we regard the change we have in mind as a process rather than a product. Where we end up is unlikely to be the place we had in mind when we started, so the process approach makes sense. As Turrill points out, 'When introducing change, the journey is at least as important as the destination' (Turrill 1986).

The experience of nurses who have already introduced model-based practice bears this out. The process of defining values, examining current practice, opening up new channels of communication and providing a fresh focus of work interest may bring at least as many benefits to nurses and patients as the final, triumphant implementation of the Heath Robinson Model for Nursing (if implementation of such a finite kind ever actually happens, which is questionable).

Let us suppose that you are a senior nurse and you wish to introduce your staff to the Heath Robinson Model, believing that it offers an appropriate framework in which they can develop their practice. How will you go about it, and how can an understanding of the process of change help you? You would be well advised to begin by heeding the wise words of Machiavelli (in Turrill 1986):

'There is nothing more difficult, more perilous to conduct, or more uncertain in its success, than to take the lead in a new order of things, because the innovator has for enemies all those who have done well under the old conditions, and lukewarm defenders in those who may do well under the new.'

Machiavelli's insight has stood the test of time. The vested interests he refers to are a fact of life – we all have them. Furthermore, people who are under great stress may be enemies to innovation even when they have not done well under the old conditions. Such people become blockers who severely limit the organisation's capacity for change. The stress factors people commonly name include conflicting demands, changing priorities, changes in the nature of their work, and major policy shifts. All these stressors are likely to occur in changing to a new kind of nursing practice. And when the overall environment is seen as insecure, as the NHS is today, people are even less able or willing to cope with change.

Put yourself in the shoes of the sister on one of the wards where you would like to introduce the model. A qualified, experienced nurse who believes she has worked well in that post for ten years is now being urged to change her ways, and perhaps to relinquish some of her authority. Shock, withdrawal and apathy are among the responses the unwary manager may provoke in her when she breezes in with her bright new idea. To what extent are they inevitable aspects of human behaviour, and to what extent can they be anticipated and controlled? Forewarned is forearmed, as Pearson and Vaughan (1986) have pointed out: 'Some changes occur because of things around us, but most changes cannot effectively occur without being planned. Planned change is inevitably easier to manage than change which is imposed, haphazard or misunderstood.'

Pearson and Vaughan advocate the use of the nursing process logic – assessment, planning, implementation and evaluation – as one way of tackling change. More broadly, the change process has been outlined as devising an overall strategy, turning it into a plan, seeking sanction from those in authority, and implementing the plan. The problem with such approaches, according to Turrill, is that people are simply not rational and these linear processes rarely work. Successful change programmes are far more complex, and more bitty. He identifies seven common features which can be worked on and which increase the likelihood of a successful, stabilised transition. Working through each of these features can provide the means to tackle it by clarifying what exactly it is you want to do. If you ignore any of these factors you are likely to face even greater obstacles.

- *Agreeing the core purposes of the organisation.* This is a crucial starting point. We may all think we agree about the core purpose of the NHS, for example, but such an assumption is dangerous and probably unfounded. The core purpose is often defined in a 'mission statement' containing the basic reasons for the organisation's existence. The wise manager would be well advised to start by encouraging her staff to identify the unit/ward/clinic's core purpose. This is the final reference point that binds them together and steers them through the chaos of change.

- *Sharing a vision of a better future.* This is the powerhouse of change: looking ahead and describing what you would like to be doing in, say, five years. Lasting change will not occur unless a critical mass of people share the vision.

For example, what specific improvements in care do you hope to achieve through model-based practice?

● *Operating principles.* These are the organisational values that help to guide the individual nurse when she is faced with uncertainty. They may state the obvious but are none the less important. For example, it may be agreed that all staff should understand and uphold the principle that care should be planned jointly with patients.

● *Mapping the environment.* A change in nursing practice will have implications for many other groups, individuals and systems, any of which could try to block change. It is crucial to identify these other domains: not all of them can be handled, so select the most important and work out how to respond to them. For example, plans should be discussed with medical staff and agreement reached on their introduction.

● *Transition management.* This highlights the need to manage the state between where you are starting out and where you want to end up; it is often neglected, but needs managing, work, resources and time. It involves defining the work required in making the change in order to allocate adequate resources to it – such as a project team, a new post, or time (whose?) to develop new care plans.

● *Resistance reduction.* Two-way communication and genuine involvement are essential to reduce the resistance to change outlined earlier. Resistance may also lie within the system; formal arrangements can be tackled, but perhaps more difficult are the informal power groupings. For example, nursing auxiliaries have little formal power but their opposition could sabotage the project. They should be involved and persuaded of the benefits.

● *Seeking commitment.* This is an essential ingredient. Identify key people and groups, and devise non-threatening ways of winning them over. New reward systems and education opportunities can help, as can a celebration when the team attains a key objective.

Using this type of framework to think about how you can plan and manage change is a helpful way of focusing ideas. Remembering that the journey to change is as important as the destination, carrying out these activities will benefit you and your staff, even if you finally decide that the Heath Robinson Model of Nursing is not, after all, the answer to your problems!

There is general agreement in the literature that leadership is central to successful change. One reasearch-based study of why some NHS innovations diffused rapidly while others were completely blocked pinpoints the key role of the change agent (Stocking 1985). The presence or absence of a product champion – a person or group who champion an idea through research and development to its final introduction – was important in determining whether the innovation was taken up. The innovators needed adequate status and drive for the job in hand, and the backing of supporters or facilitators, who were often managers.

The manager, then, may not necessarily be the leader or champion, but can play a vital back-room role. This distinction may be worth considering in your own team so that roles can be tailored to individual competencies and potential. The leadership role may be adopted for a particular project, just as the leadership of the multidisciplinary team can be conceptualised as a role that different team members may adopt at different times.

Creating a climate in which leaders can emerge and innovation is encouraged is one of the manager's key functions. Management style is very important. It does not depend on structures (though structures do have implications for style), but on how the manager goes about her job. Again this is just as relevant to the ward sister as it is to the unit manager. Do staff participate in goal-setting and other strategic activities? Does every person feel valued and are their accomplishments recognised? How is the manager perceived and how are their priorities viewed? We would like to feel that nursing is moving in the right direction, but there is still a long way to go. From the bottom looking up, the main impression is still one of large numbers of unseen senior people issuing orders which are passed down the line; those at the bottom have little direct contact with those above sister, and that contact still tends to be overwhelmingly negative.

The successful introduction of a nursing model, or of any other change, is unlikely to occur unless your part of the organisation is one that fosters innovation and exploration of all kinds. When that spirit is prevalent, the question of Heath Robinson's model is seen not as a major one-off event, but as just one of a whole range of possible changes. In an organisation which is innovative rather than conservative, change is seen as more normal and less shocking; indeed as a way of life. This is clearly the experience of nurses in settings that have become a byword for innovation, such as the nursing development units at Oxford and Tameside (Pearson 1988, Wright 1986).

When examining the work of these units, it is hard to nominate one single change as the key to their success. Was it the introduction of model-based practice, primary nursing, or a flattening of the hierarchical structure that was most crucial? Perhaps the key was the commitment of most staff – nurses and others – to put the needs and wishes of each patient at the centre of their work; a precept often preached but less often practised. Probably, though, it was none of these factors in isolation, but a continuing desire to explore and try out new ideas. This sense of exploration may in itself be the major change successfully introduced by the nurses.

This need to transform nursing into a culture in which change is a way of life should be a prime motive for promoting model-based practice. If your own part of the organisation is conservative rather than innovative, models is a good topic with which to start the transformation, because it gets right to the heart of what nursing is about. Models make people think, and anything that makes nurses think about nursing is worth support. McFarlane (1986) warns that 'models may become just another fashion because of the inability of nurses to integrate them into a creative and innovative approach to nursing practice'. But she concludes more hopefully: 'The profession needs to accept the present lively debate [about models] as a challenge to explore our practice and to liberate ourselves from the assumption that there is a right and uniform way to nurse.'

References

Kershaw B & Salvage J, eds (1986) *Models for Nursing.* Chichester: John Wiley.

McFarlane J (1986) Looking to the future. In Kershaw B & Salvage J, eds. *Models for Nursing.* Chichester: John Wiley.

Pearson A, ed. (1988) *Primary Nursing.* London: Croom Helm.

Pearson A & Vaughan B (1986) *Nursing Models for Practice.* London: Heinemann.

Stocking B (1985) *Initiative and Inertia: Case Studies in the NHS.* London: Nuffield Provincial Hospitals Trust.

Turrill T (1986) *Change and Innovation: A Challenge for the NHS.* Management Series 10, London: Institute of Health Services Management.

Wright S (1986) *Building and Using a Model of Nursing.* London: Edward Arnold.

Models for Nursing 2
Edited by B Kershaw and J Salvage
© 1990 Scutari Press

2

A Critical Perspective

PAUL CHAPMAN

'Recently there has been extensive adoption of theoretical frameworks or models in the nursing profession. Schools of nursing, hospitals, community health units – many profess to be using one or other of the models. Worryingly there is little resistance in the literature to this kind of "blanket adoption". The lack of criticism, or comment, in a field which is claiming to have arrived in the scientific world, but which is not yet established, may be damning evidence to the true state of nursing as a profession.' – HARDY, 1986

This chapter is based on the work of the dissenting minority who offer resistance to the 'blanket adoption' of nursing models – writers with the audacity to challenge officially sanctioned views about the value of nursing theory and nursing models. This received wisdom centres around the belief that nursing needs to establish itself as a unique and independent profession by developing its own theoretical base, scientifically organised around a conceptual framework ('model'), and assumes that such a development will benefit patients as well as the 'profession'.

The strength of this official position is not to be underestimated. Wright (1985) referred to the active encouragement of model development by the English National Board for Nursing, Midwifery and Health Visiting, while Johnson (1986) felt unable to criticise a series of articles on models without assuring the authors that he was not attacking them personally. He paints a sorry picture of how rigorous academic criticism is stifled in nursing: 'Academics trained in the much harsher but more realistic worlds of the natural sciences and perhaps sociology are shocked by the obvious back-slapping and "hear hear" attitude which prevails at nursing research conferences. Asking a searching question of a speaker at such an event is seen as terribly bad form – even worse form should the speaker be one of the eminent (Johnson 1986, p. 42).'

On first examination, the numerous references to lack of agreement and clarity of terminology in nursing theory might be regarded as evidence of the healthy debate which Johnson and others suggest is lacking. However, the mainstream literature has tended not to question the tenets outlined above, but has concerned itself with clarifying such terms as 'theory', 'model' and 'conceptual framework'. Some writers consider 'theory' and 'model' to be synonymous, some differentiate absolutely between the two, and some take a position somewhere in between. This lack of precision about basic terms is hardly appropriate for a would-be scientific discipline, and Newman (1979) goes as far as suggesting that the terms are often so vague that they have little meaning (p.5).

For present purposes the term 'nursing theory' will be used as a convenient global term to incorporate the work on nursing models, in keeping with the view of Weatherstone (1979) that model building can be considered as paradigmatic theory. Similarly, academic work on the nursing process is included here under the umbrella of 'nursing theory'. The term 'nursing model' is here intended to mean any set of concepts called a model by its author; consideration of whether a model is a model, and according to whose definition, will be eschewed for the moment.

Medical *versus* nursing models

The case for adopting nursing models rests partly on the assertion that nursing care should not be based on theories borrowed from other disciplines, particularly medicine. The word 'borrowed' is significant, with its negative connotations of an unsatisfactory transience, and the 'theory shopping' approach is compared unfavourably with the development of unique, specific nursing science to form the cornerstone of an independent profession. As Clark (1982) puts it, 'any attempt to construct a model of nursing, *however poor and inadequate the model may turn out to be,* makes explicit the notion that there is something called nursing which has an identity of its own, distinct from other similar activities ... The universal acceptance of the independent identity of nursing would be a tremendous leap forward in the development of nursing as a profession' (my italics).

Clark advances her argument by suggesting that those who find nursing models unacceptable are 'people (including some nurses) who still see nursing merely as a collection of tasks on the initiation of and under the direction of doctors' (p.131). Thus criticism of the medical model (on which nursing is still perceived as dependent) leads to the apparently logical conclusion that what nursing needs is its own model which, it is implied, will be superior. As Hardy (1982) observes, 'Riehl and Roy cast a critical eye on the medical model which they saw as narrowing. The same critical eye was not turned on nursing because it seemed that the profession was one up on the doctors. That is, nursing's emphasis is on patients, not diseases' (p.449).

Criticism of the medical model and the medical profession may well be justified. Hardy's point, however, is that 'one track is one track, however defined'. That is, it is not desirable to replace one élitist, restricting perspective with another. She says that nursing models have been created 'to bestow respectability and credibility upon our profession. This is in response to how other professions have evolved. Perhaps it is time to question ... whether or not professions utilizing models have served the public well ... Professionalizing helps to define, to set apart. This includes the use of semantic confusion and élitist ideas' (p.106).

Cronenwett (1983) also challenges the assertion that professionalising by means of developing nursing models is inherently good for patient care. Furthermore, this author finds similarities between medical and nursing models: 'The medical model [assumes] that people cannot be expected to solve their problems. The help recipient, viewed as sick, is expected to get well by seeking and using expert help ... Half of the nursing models and definitions reviewed contained statements that implied nurses use a medical-model approach to helping' (p.343).

The point here is that whether someone is seen as 'sick' or 'at some point on a health–illness continuum', as having a 'diseased sub-system' or as a 'bio-psychosocial being', the issue is essentially semantic if in reality one expert who diagnoses and controls (the doctor) is merely replaced by another (the nurse). Cronenwett thus looks behind the terminology of models such as Orem and Roy and questions whether the patient-centred approaches described are a facade: 'Is the whole idea of mutually established goals just a polite way of saying that the provider manipulates the client into agreeing with the provider's solutions? ... the problem the patient brings to the situation is usually reformulated by the expert prior to the problem-solving ... Is any model of helping effective if the problem is defined solely by the helper?' (p.345).

Perhaps, then, we should not take it as read that the professionalising of nursing is inevitably good for patient care. The term 'professional' is over-used in nursing, and it is pertinent to note Katz's statement that few professionals talk as much about being professionals as those whose professional status is in doubt (1969, p.71). It is also interesting to analyse what makes the label such a desirable one. Gruending (1985) lists monopoly of service, autonomy, public recognition, prestige, power, authority, as well as monetary and status rewards, as the goodies on offer. Moreover, the professionalising process is inextricably linked with the development of a discrete terminology which serves to 'increase mystique, thereby decreasing the public's comprehension of what is involved in nursing' (Gruending 1985). Hardy (1986) links this distancing of nurse and patient directly with model development: 'Models promote the use of specialised concepts and jargon which necessitate lengthy orientation, a procedure which is not available to health consumers; thus a distance is created between carer and consumer, and between professions' (p.103).

Research validating nursing theories and models

How much hard, research-based evidence exists in the nursing theory debate? 'Few nurses were without grave reservations about nursing theories ... It now seems to be considered pretentious to dignify these frameworks with lofty names when they amount to no more than a collection of unverified assumptions which reflect the personal philosophies or value-systems of their authors', Webb claims

84). The lack of research to validate nursing theories and models has been lamented subsequent to Webb's stinging article by, among others, Green (1985) and Hardy (1986). These criticisms have gone unchallenged, however, because the research on which nursing should be based (according to the orthodox view) does not exist to support nursing models. Instead we are given case studies illustrating the model in use, often describing it in enthusiastic terms but making no attempt to validate it through rigorous methodology (see, for example, Barker 1984, Campbell 1984, Dyer 1985).

Roper, Logan and Tierney (1983) commissioned nine such case studies for a textbook, in order to 'test the authors' belief that the nursing model described in the previous two books is a conceptual framework which can be used in any health care setting'. The contributors were not randomly selected, but hand-picked on the grounds of having 'sufficient individuality to think through their actions, analyse their actions and reactions, then write about the experience'. The authors note that there was considerable enthusiasm for the project, and armed with this enthusiasm and a copy of *The Elements of Nursing* (1980) given to them at a meeting with editors and publisher, the contributors set about their task. Some nit-picking apart, each contributor declares the model to be useful and is keen for more. This methodology hardly constitutes scientific research, nor does it justify the rather grandiose claims often made for the model (although it is undoubtedly one of the simplest and most comprehensible).

There is a more serious defence of this lack of validating research which must also be addressed. The assertion is that conceptual models are valuable not as testable theories but as a 'preparadigm' stage of scientific development, as described by Kuhn (1970). According to this analysis it is less important whether the model is called a theory; its rationale is its ability to provide a broad, abstract framework describing relationships between concepts (a 'world view' or para-digm) from which can emerge testable hypotheses 'specifying relations among variables derived from these ideas' (Fawcett 1980). Chance (1982) supports this analysis, and emphasises that the model must generate tools and hypotheses that can be empirically analysed through research in order to satisfy the criterion of usefulness.

Persuasive as this argument might be in deflecting criticism of the lack of validating research, a crucial question must nevertheless be asked: where are the specific, testable hypotheses meant to emerge from these conceptual frameworks? There is precious little evidence of such emergence, as Crow (1982) asserts; one obvious conclusion is that the models do not in fact stimulate readily testable hypotheses. Hardy is less hasty, however, preferring the explanation that 'energy [is] going into attempts to justify one of several embryonic paradigms rather than into purposeful orderly research' (1978). Unfortunately, exactly the same point was made in 1982 and 1986, so it appears that little progress is being made.

The clinical nurse attempting to use a nursing model is therefore faced with broad concepts, which do not prescribe nursing actions for specific situations, as Chenitz and Swanson (1984) point out. This is exacerbated by the fact that many of the models claim universal applicability in an occupation which is becoming increasingly specialised and diversified. Moreover, it is suggested, the claim that nursing models are a discrete contrast to the 'borrowed' medical model is disingenuous, as many of the individual concepts within the frameworks are 'borrowed' from other disciplines. Another problem the would-be implementer might face is identified by Miller, who says that nursing theorists are concerned with 'nursing as it ought to be' and not 'as it is' (1985).

Nursing as science

As suggested earlier, the development of nursing theory is perceived as a move towards science and away from ritualistic traditions. However, the philosophical assumptions that underlie different perspectives on science comprise an area of study all of their own. The embracing of a particular scientific rationale is a deep and complex issue, but all too often such analysis is lacking in writings on nursing theory.

Although Nightingale is sometimes described as the first nurse theorist, attempts to develop nursing as a science have been slow and arduous. In Britain, the attraction of the academicisation of nursing through empirical research has been its 'scientific' rationale, as opposed to the hide-bound, ritualistic, task-orientated approach passed unquestioningly from one generation to the next, and underpinned by subservience to doctors. Ironically, in trying to free itself from medical domination, nursing's tactics have often consisted of attempts to emulate the medical profession. This was the motivation, for example, behind the Royal College of Nursing's longstanding resistance to pay rises for students until 1948. If nursing was to emerge from the shadow of medicine, it must be perceived as being equally 'scientific'. This position, however, assumes an uncritical, restricted view of science: that it is by definition good, and that scientific research leads to objective knowledge.

Doyal (1979) describes the relationship between science and medicine which many theorists seek to establish for nursing: 'First, it is assumed that the determinants of health and illness are predominantly biological, so that patterns of morbidity and mortality have little to do with the social and economic environment in which they occur. As a consequence ... broader ideas of social change are seen as largely irrelevant ... and medical progress is said to be based on the use of "scientific" method which supposedly ensures certain and objective knowledge. Hence it is usually believed that medicine, because it is "scientific", can produce an unchallengeable and autonomous body of knowledge which is not tainted by wider social and economic considerations' (p.12).

But surely, the cry goes up, many nursing models emphasise the importance of psychological and social aspects of health, and advocate patients' involvement in their care? This is true of some of the theory, but in practice such aims easily become little more than the inclusion of a section of the care plan for 'social and psychological' aspects. Problems are assessed and diagnosed by the nurse expert, with only token attempts to embrace patient autonomy, because the very concept of the omniscient professional works against democratic involvment by the patient. A 'scientific' profession depends on restricted access to its body of knowledge and the maintenance of mystique which eschews open communication. Far from offering radical alternatives to the medical model, nursing models tend to criticise certain aspects of it but retain an analysis of science and health rooted in sociological functionalism (see my own critique of Orem's model, Chapman 1984). Even models that claim an interactionist approach seek to present 'nursing' as something pure and objective rather than a product of the society in which it takes place.

A further question must be asked: if the arguments for nursing models are so overwhelming, why do nurses need to be manipulated or coerced into using them? A more 'scientific' and ethical approach would be to hold study sessions incorporating open-minded discussion, when clinical nurses, managers and teachers could decide for themselves whether a particular nursing model merited experimental implementation. This is the approach adopted in the care of the elderly unit at Tameside General Hospital. Eschewing 'the imposition of an established model as if from God on high', Wright and his fellow joint-appointee worked with clinical nurses in a facilitating role; 'much effort was needed to avoid the impression of something being imposed from above ... Our initial steps involved meetings – lots of them, just talking about nursing and asking questions. The first was inevitably, "What do we believe nursing to be?" It took at least four months to pull together a ward philosophy' (Wright 1985).

Lewin (1945) suggests that democratic, group decision-making is far more effective in implementing meaningful change than an authoritarian, dictatorial approach. Unfortunately it is the latter which appears to flourish in nursing. I underestimated the capacity of the nursing establishment to impose change from above when I speculated that there was little prospect of the implementation of new nursing theories being anything other than sporadic (Chapman 1984). More recent experience has shown that nursing models are introduced in ways closer to 'imposition' than to 'implementation'.

Wright (1985) has observed that difficulties may arise if the ENB's encouragement of model development in schools of nursing is interpreted rigidly. Nurse teachers and managers, whilst they may express private doubts, feel obliged in public to support the use of nursing models. Speculatively, the motives for this may be related to the idea that they ought to be given a try on the wards; or there may be an element of competition as nursing models replace nursing process as the hallmark of a progressive, dynamic hospital. Instead of the democratic Tameside approach, it is possible that the following is more usual: senior nurses and tutors decide which model will be used in each ward or unit, and charge nurses and staff are requested to become acquainted with it (with varying amounts of help from the school and service side) and to interpret and use it on their ward. Enthusiasm for the project may understandably be grudging, so the minimum is done to satisfy the requirements. Journal articles (especially those of Aggleton & Chalmers 1984), which are simplifications of the original models, are further simplified to be of practical use – with the exception of the Roper, Logan and Tierney model, which hardly needs any simplification. The care plans are reorganised accordingly, and may be displayed to any visiting dignitary. The actual changes to patient care need not be studied (by, for example, establishing control groups) as honour has already been satisfied all round.

Future prospects

This chapter has deliberately been based on the work of writers who, from various standpoints, are critical of the blanket adoption of nursing models. If, in Hegelian terms, the emergence of their work can be seen as the antithesis to the pro-models thesis, what then will be the synthesis or resolution? Silva and Rothbart (1984) are optimistic, based on their discernment of a trend in nursing theory away from logical empiricism and towards historicism: 'Based on this historicist orientation, there should not be a single conceptual framework for nursing. This orientation suggests, rather, the expansion of nursing theory through the integration of pro-gressive components of the various existing nursing conceptual frameworks, which results in multiple frameworks. This process should be a co-operative endeavour and, if adhered to, should encourage a co-operative rather than a competitive attitude among nurse scholars. In the future some of the conceptual frameworks for nursing may be integrated so that the unimportant elements are sacrificed and the important elements are combined in a new way' (p 11).

This cosy co-operation of rival theorists may be hard to imagine, but it is easier to accept that nursing models are here to stay. More criticisms may yet emerge, but nursing is an occupation historically dominated by powerful élites, and the evidence suggests that today's leaders are firmly behind the concept of nursing models. There are two positive ways of viewing this, both fallacious. The first is that such force from the top is necessary to ensure change in an occupation notoriously resistant to it – but it may be that the change that results is nowhere near as meaningful as is claimed, because people who have not been convinced of its value merely do the minimum necessary to satisfy their superiors. Even in units where the care plans are up to standard, the care might not necessarily have improved accordingly; nurses may now find themselves forced to reorganise the care plans again, this time around a nursing model, but life will carry on very much as before.

The second fallacy is that there is no harm in experimenting with nursing models, so why not try. This ignores the potential damage of elevating the unique status of nursing above the concept of the multidisciplinary team; for example, it has implications for the psychotherapeutic role developments evolving in psychiatric nursing. In addition, time and energy spent on nursing models might be better spent on other issues – although if front-line nurses have genuine interest and enthusiasm for models, no-one should dictate that they do anything than pursue that interest.

Fellow nurses often seem to find my interest in nursing models rather perplex-ing. The usual response is lack of interest, tinged with guilt about lack of know-ledge about what is clearly a vogue concept. My hope is that a more critical approach will develop and flourish, representing a far superior, truly professional approach: independent-minded practitioners making their own judgements, based on rational argument and evidence, with the tangible, immediate needs of recipients and givers of nursing care firmly in mind.

References

Aggleton P & Chalmers H (1984) Models and theories. Series in *Nursing Times*, **80,** 5 September 1984 to **81,** 3 April 1985.

Barker J (1984) A plan for Arthur and Mary. *Nursing Times,* **80,** *Community Outlook,* 403–408.

Campbell C (1984) Orem's story. *Nursing Mirror,* **151**(13), 28–30.

Chance K (1982) Nursing models: a requisite for professional accountability. *Advances in Nursing Science,* January, 57–65.

Chapman P (1984) Specifics and generalities: a critical examination of two nursing models. *Nurse Education Today,* **4**(6), 141–144.

Chenitz C & Swanson J (1984) Surfacing nursing process: a method for generating nursing theory from practice. *Journal of Advanced Nursing,* **9**(2), 205–215.

Clark J (1982) Development of models and theories on the concept of nursing. *Journal of Advanced Nursing,* **7**(2), 129–134.

Cronenwett L (1983) Helping and nursing models. *Nursing Research,* **32**(6), 342–346.

Crow R (1982) Frontiers of nursing in the 21st century: development of models and theories on the concept of nursing. *Journal of Advanced Nursing,* **7**(2), 111–116.

Doyal L (1979) *The Political Economy of Health.* London: Pluto Press.

Dyer J (1985) A model of care. *Nursing Mirror,* 24 April, 28–30.

Fawcett J (1980) A framework for analysis and evaluation of conceptual models of nursing. *Nurse Educator,* **5**(6), 10–14.

Green C (1985) An overview of the value of nursing models in relation to education. *Nurse Education Today,* **5**(6), 267–271.

Gruending D (1985) Nursing theory: a vehicle for professionalisation? *Journal of Advanced Nursing,* **10**(6), 553–558.

Hardy L (1982) Nursing models and research – a restricting view? *Journal of Advanced Nursing,* **7**(5), 447–451.

Hardy L (1986) Identifying the place of theoretical frameworks in an evolving discipline. *Journal of Advanced Nursing,* **11**(1), 103–107.

Hardy M (1978) Perspectives on nursing theory. *Advances in Nursing Science,* **1,** 37–48.

Johnson M (1986) Model of perfection. *Nursing Times,* **82**(5), 42–43.

Katz F (1969) Nurses. In Etzioni A, ed, *The Semi-Professions and their Organisations.* USA: Free Press.

Kuhn T (1970) *The Structure of Scientific Revolutions.* Chicago: University of Chicago Press.

Lewin K (1945) *Group Decisions and Social Change.* Washington, DC: US Government Research Department.

Miller A (1985) The relationship between nursing theory and nursing practice. *Journal of Advanced Nursing,* **10**(5), 417–424.

Newman M (1979) *Theory Development in Nursing.* Philadelphia: Davis.

Roper N, Logan W & Tierney A (1980) *The Elements of Nursing.* Edinburgh: Churchill Livingstone.

Roper N, Logan W & Tierney A (1983) *Using a Model for Nursing.* Edinburgh: Churchill Livingstone.

Silva M & Rothbart D (1984) An analysis of changing trends in philosophies of science on nursing theory development and testing. *Advances in Nursing Science,* **6**(2), 1–13.

Weatherstone L (1979) Theory of nursing: creating effective care. *Journal of Advanced Nursing,* **4,** 365–375.

Webb C (1984) On the eighth day God created the nursing process and nobody rested. *Senior Nurse,* **1**(33), 22–25.

Wright S (1985) Strategy for change. *Senior Nurse*, **3**(4) October, 24–25.

Models for Nursing 2
Edited by B Kershaw and J Salvage
© 1990 Scutari Press

3

Useless Theory or Aid to Practice?

STEVE WRIGHT

This chapter explores some of the current issues related to the debate on nursing models. It examines some of the advantages and problems, and suggests how model-based practice can be developed using a 'bottom-up' strategy involving and led by nurses at clinical level.

Towards coherence in practice

Quite simply, a model may be regarded as being a combination of:

- how the individual nurse perceives nursing;
- how the nurse organises his or her nursing;
- how groups of nurses think about and organise their nursing.

Reilly (1975) notes how each nurse carries in his or her head an image of what nursing is. It is the purpose of models to help bring together the images held by a variety of nurses, so that they have common goals and a shared understanding. The alternative is a lack of sense of direction, and the adoption of a multiplicity of approaches, not all of them nursing, such as where nursing subordinates itself to the disease and treatment orientation of the medical model. This leads to confusion among both patients and nurses, as Pearson and Vaughan (1986) have illustrated. During the course of a few minutes, a patient or client may encounter several nurses, each offering a different approach:

'Don't worry, I'll do everything for you.'
'Come on, you have to learn to do it for yourself.'
'I'll have to get the doctor to talk to you first.'

It is not difficult to imagine the contrasting experiences and conflicts of nurses and patients when the sister in charge one day is the rod-of-iron, doing-every-thing-for-the-patients, task-centred type, and next day the sister in charge adopts a nursing style that emphasises rehabilitation, partnership and involvement with patients. All nurses have come across these types during their nursing life. Different models can be confusing not only for patients, but also for staff.

It is a contradiction in terms to suggest that nurses do not have or do not need models of nursing. Every nurse carries that image in her head of what nursing is and, most crucially, this image determines practice – a major reason why nursing models cannot be ignored. We may not like the uncomfortable feelings involved in trying to define or clarify what nursing is and how it shall be done, but the most important factor about each nurse's model, however inexplicit, incoherent or informal, is that the nurse acts it out. The way we think about nursing determines how we do it, and nurses must think about their models of care because what they think affects patients. When models are not made explicit, shared with colleagues and based on a sound rationale and research, what nurses end up doing may not actually be nursing. Martin (1984) shows how 'care' can be corrupted to the point of abuse of patients, denial of their rights and sheer cruelty – partly arising when nurses do not share a clear vision of what nursing is or what it might be.

Details of how a nursing model can be 'acted out' have been documented else-where (Wright 1986, 1988; Purdy, Wright & Johnson 1988a), but a few factors can be summarised here. How can it be shown that the model is a reality? What is going on in the clinical setting which shows that nursing is following a particular path? There may be a noble philosophy of care pinned to the notice board, which everybody ignores, or there may be a real translation of ideas into practice. Figure 3.1 illustrates some of the factors that provide evidence of model-based practice.

A nursing model provides nurses with a frame of reference, a pattern of thoughts and actions, which enables them to make explicit the art and science of nursing. It can help them to articulate to each other, to patients and to other professions who they are and what they do – a sign of maturity in any profession. A clear identity enables the nurse to stand her ground with other members of the multidisciplinary team in promoting high-quality care. Only from a team of equals can effective multi-disciplinary care arise: if nursing is not contributing fully, the patient is short-changed and other disciplines may step in to fill the vacuum. This may be dangerous for nurses too, for if they do not define what nursing is, others will do it for them. Traditionally this has been done by doctors, and more recently by general managers. As the poet William Blake notes in *Jerusalem*, we must 'create a system or be enslaved by another man's.' Many factors have hindered nursing's power to determine its own destiny – related to gender, class, public perception and so on – but one key feature is nurses' ability to define what they do and how to do it. Relying solely on our own informal models maintains a weakness that contributes to nursing's low status. The crea-tion of more formal, explicit models is part of the process towards self-determination.

Yet, while models are part of the call for nurses to assert themselves, it should not be thought that nurses can be the sole determinants of nursing. Everybody has

Management
- Staff support meetings
- Agreement on philosophies, policies, objectives
- Open, participative climate/style of management, acting as support system to clinical nurses
- Quality assurance programme
- Managers are practitioners/clinical experts
- Management development programmes

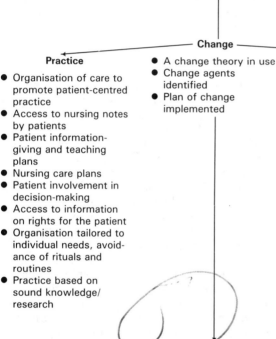

— Change —

Practice
- Organisation of care to promote patient-centred practice
- Access to nursing notes by patients
- Patient information-giving and teaching plans
- Nursing care plans
- Patient involvement in decision-making
- Access to information on rights for the patient
- Organisation tailored to individual needs, avoidance of rituals and routines
- Practice based on sound knowledge/research

- A change theory in use
- Change agents identified
- Plan of change implemented

Education
- Individual staff development plans
- Ongoing, on-site courses, conferences, seminars
- Support/funding for time off
- Open learning climate
- Teachers as practitioners
- Learning opportunities for all staff
- On-site access to literature, journals etc.

Research
- Research-based practice
- Individual/group activity carrying out research
- Implementation of findings
- Acceptance of research activity, atmosphere of enquiry
- Staff with specific brief to support/carry out research
- Publishing of activities/research

Figure 3.1 The model in action – some possible factors as evidence (after Wright (1988) and Purdy, Wright and Johnson (1988a, b))

a theory of nursing – other disciplines, relatives and patients – and nurses must work with and take account of these views. Most importantly, it is the patient who must determine practice; the consumer of care, armed with the right to make informed choices, must determine what sort of nursing is desired. All nursing models must therefore incorporate quality assurance or evaluation of care by patients and their informal carers. Working in partnership with patients and others, taking account of and testing their views and constantly reviewing prac-tice is an essential counterbalance to the development of nursing along the traditional professional road; nurses should not become part of George Bernard Shaw's 'conspiracy against the laity' by being élitist, exclusive and self-serving. They should not exercise power over patients, but should be powerful with them. Sharing knowledge and skill in caring is essential to empower the patient and informal carers to achieve self-determination. Nursing is a service *for* patients, but it must also be a service *with* patients.

Ivory tower or coalface?

Models, then, may help but they are not panaceas. They will not cure nursing ills overnight. However, if the current media debate is anything to go by, they have at least stirred up further argument and discussion about nursing (e.g. Johnson 1985, Lister 1987, Luker 1988). This might sometimes be painful, but it shows that nursing is alive and kicking. Argument is a sign of health – without it there is little but dull conformity.

Cautionary, even hostile comments about nursing models have regularly appeared in the nursing press recently. Dylak (1986) writes of 'nursing model fever' and expresses reservations about the validity of the underlying assumptions of many models, often unproven; he fears they may be imposed on nurses, with a consequent reaction against them. Johnson (1985) meanwhile argues that there has been 'a good deal more conjecture than refutation', with many writings on models being 'wholly uncritical'. He too is concerned that nurse managers or educators may select one model and blindly apply it to their curriculum or clinical practice. Luker (1988) suggests that models might be red herrings, inappropriate to nursing, which divert attention from other areas of activity.

Sternberg (1986), as a student nurse, rejects the notion that nursing models could help to change practice: 'I have recently been trying to get to grips with nursing models by following a well-thought-out and researched learning package. It occurred to me, while wrestling with the Roy model, that even if I did understand it, it would make no difference to the way I actually nurse. It might help me to write a nursing care plan or an essay in my finals but it will not change the way I nurse in the ward.' Models are seen as unrealistic because they are said to represent the views of a minority of 'academic nurses'; they strive to be all-embracing about nursing knowledge and practice but 'in trying to explain everything, they may explain nothing' (Miller 1985).

Webb (1984) argues that it seems 'pretentious to dignify these frameworks with names where they amount to no more than a collection of unverified assumptions which reflect the personal philosophies or value systems of their authors'. Graham (1987) suggests that the recent advocacy of models produces ridicule and rejection among some clinical nurses and educators, because of the alienating language and the apparent pretentiousness: 'Terminologies such as "disruptive wellness", "repatterned energy fields", "significant life crises" may be meat and drink to the sociologists and psychologists among nurse teachers. But to the majority of clinical nurses, it is an affront to their intelligence. As the model designers go from systems to interactions to energy fields to behaviours to adaptions, the front line troops are beginning to revolt. And ridicule is a very potent weapon.'

In some respects the result has been to produce yet another theory and practice gap. Nursing models, for all the richness and value they can bring, may end up remote from practice – esoteric notions that keep the ivory tower nurse happy, but fail to reach the coalface of nursing.

Currently, it could be argued, nursing is intellectually and practically in a state of confusion. Gaps between theory and practice, research and practice, management and education, and many other factors have led to a diversity of approaches which at best leave nurses confused and at worst are harmful to patients. Lessons should be drawn from the past in introducing nursing models. The danger of creating another theory–practice gap is illustrated by the introduction of the nursing process in the UK. This change was characterised by four fatal flaws (Wright 1986), which led to confusion, hostility and rejection, persisting in many areas to this day. An excellent nursing ideal suffered because:

- It was seen as being imposed from above, e.g. by teachers or managers who were not perceived as practitioners.
- There was a lack of adequate preparation and education.
- There was too little support for nurses changing to a new approach.
- Nurses were asked to use the process before nursing had clearly defined its role.

It could be argued, indeed, that nursing tried to put the cart before the horse – to rethink nursing when there was little shared perception of what nursing was; that is, no clear nursing models. Thus nurses often tried to apply the nursing process to their traditional, medical-model thinking – but the two do not fit comfortably together.

The importance of planning change

Many of the conflicts surrounding nursing models are characteristic of the process of change in general. We need to learn the lesson of the nursing process that top-down strategies will never work for nursing models; they lead to misunderstanding, to rejection and reaction, to models being seen as new forms of paperwork instead of a contribution to creative practice. Otherwise we will hear those classic markers of ineffective change: 'Oh, we're not using the model tonight because we're short-staffed,' or 'We don't bother when sister is off duty'. A clearly mapped change strategy must accompany any development of nursing models.

It is worth noting at this point that developing nursing models opens a can of worms in terms of the kind of education and management needed by model-using nurses. A different breed of nurse needs a different kind of educa-tion and management. One of the problems with the nursing process, for example, was a lack of understanding of what would happen if nurses were weaned away from task allocation. Menzies (1961) had indicated that tasks were a shield to protect nurses from the anxiety of total involvement with patients – for which they were traditionally ill-prepared and ill-supported. When the props of task allocation were taken away, were they replaced with other means of support? Were nurses offered the communication skills, problem-solving skills and coping mechanisms they needed to survive? Another test of a nursing model is how far it replaces one set of props with another, or leaves the nurse adrift in a sea of change without support. With the nursing process, it seems that these vital coping strategies were not replaced. The nurse who uses a model is an expert, creative, questioning nurse who needs a different education and manage-ment strategy to produce and support her.

Nursing models may be classified according to how far they encompass some significant areas of thought. They should have something to say about the follow-ing major concepts:

● the nature of the person and his or her environment;
● the concept of health;
● the concept of nursing;

and how each overlaps with the others. A model should also offer guidelines on:

● what kind of research is relevant to nursing;
● how nursing should be managed to produce creative practice;
● the content and style of educational programmes needed to produce the knowledgeable, problem-solving thinker;
● guidelines for the conduct of nursing practice to produce high-quality care.

Do all models do this? Many omit large areas of detail; above all, there is a great deal of emphasis on the need to change practice, but a lack of advice on how this may be done. This is crucial to the movement from one approach to nursing to another. Change, to a greater or lesser degree, will occur in any setting where a nursing model is adopted. The model should therefore have something to say about change and how it can be achieved.

Nursing tends to use the power-coercive approach, imposing change through the hierarchy. This is inappropriate if nurses are also expected to be questioning and creative (as all models require). The change must be from the bottom up (Ottaway 1976, Wright 1986, Pearson and Vaughan 1986), involving an on-site change agent to work with clinical nurses, helping them, supporting them and taking account of their views. Nurses need to feel comfortable with models, so it is necessary to start from where they are. If models are simply imposed, the 'shifting sand' effect will occur. A nurse may implement change, but when she moves on the place reverts to its old norms, like footprints in the wet sand of the beach filling up as you walk on: looking back, the footprints are filled and nothing has changed.

For new norms to become accepted and permanent there must be input from those who use them; everyone has something to contribute. Those who are to use the model need to feel they 'own' it by being party to its creation. In doing so they will adhere to its ideals long after the guiding light of the change agent has moved on. Otherwise the model may be seen as a transient theory, used when the boss is there, but not when he/she isn't!

Some would argue that 'average' clinical nurses do not have the intellect or skills to build a nursing model. My experience shows that given the necessary help – such as interaction with an on-site, knowledgeable change agent – their achievements can be astounding. The 'grounded theory' approach to nursing models (Chenitz & Swanson 1985) is probably the best option for producing real long-term change. Other approaches, like the current exhortations of the English National Board for Nursing, Midwifery and Health Visiting that schools of nursing should use a model-based curriculum, expose nurses to the danger of having a model imposed on them with all the accompanying problems of rejection and resistance. In the eagerness to develop model-based practice, are some people being forced to accept a particular model? It is better for the nurse to be offered a choice, being given:

- a variety of nursing models to choose from;
- education to help make a realistic choice;
- support from manager/educator/change agent to help with the choice and provide expertise;
- the ability and authority to modify/develop the model as new knowledge and needs emerge.

Nurses are quite capable of building their own model (Wright 1986) and, perhaps most importantly, describing it in their own language. The need to refer to American texts is questionable, since their language is alienating, they are derived from a different culture, and their assumptions are often unproven or based on different values.

Another key element of a model is its openness. A model cannot afford to reduce nursing to a fixed, tunnel-vision approach, yet nurses may still feel less comfortable or secure with an open approach; not everyone feels free to have their ideas challenged in a state of slow, continuous revolution. 'Sometimes it is safer to be in chains than to be free', as Kafka wrote. For example, in our development of a model at Tameside (Wright 1986), the move towards primary nursing was underestimated, as was the potential of the nurse's role as partner with patients, and of drawing complementary therapies into nursing practice. This is not to advocate anarchy, but an acknowledgement that knowledge is constantly expanding and nursing models need to be receptive to it. A nursing model must be open to new ideas, prepared to test them out, and ready to reject outmoded ones.

Testing the model's values

It should be possible to evaluate the nursing activity guided by the model. Does the nurse's work make life better for her patients and for herself? What values are used to decide what is 'better'? There is a danger in models that the nurse may impose her own values on the patients, but she is not always right, and the patient may not always agree. A report in *Nursing Standard* (1987), noting the results of a survey, said that only 5% of women responding would be happy if a nurse rather than a doctor was their first point of contact; just 6% said they would seek health education from a health visitor. 'Clearly nurses have some way to go to achieve the status they would like to have. The message from far too many is "You are great as long as you stay in your place and are kind to us"', it concluded.

Everybody has a theory of nursing, including the patient, whose definition of 'good' nursing may not always coincide with the nurse's. Partnership through quality assurance must underpin all nursing models, so that nurses explain to patients everything they do. Failures in communication of this type lead to many of the complaints investigated by the health service ombudsman.

Most 'modellers' agree that the philosophy stated, shared and agreed by on-site nurses is a model's most crucial feature. From this, all further development grows. Does the nursing model have a philosophy? Do colleagues share it? What are its underlying values and do they fit with nurses' and patients' views of the world? Since everybody has a theory of nursing, nurses need to be theoretical pluralists to take on board the complex issues this raises. Nursing is by nature an eclectic science and art, so an eclectic approach to theories and models is needed. Indeed, the eclecticism of nursing, its ability to take on and use knowledge from many fields, may be one of its greatest strengths.

Language is another important issue. Many theorists, particularly those from the USA, use terms alien and confusing to many British nurses. However, it is the role of the change agent to help nurses see beyond this and to interpret them if necessary, so nurses can discover the useful concepts buried within. It is debatable whether nursing should be expressed in such terms in the first place: although there is nothing wrong with new language, which is inevitably itself subject to change, we may question why the theory is expressed in a certain way. Is it genuinely using new words to express new ideas for which old words are inadequate, and does it help understanding of the model, or is the language used to gain academic respectability or to assert the theorist's superiority over the common run of nurses? Despite Graham's (1987) reservations, there are now plenty of texts in plain English. Roper, Logan and Tierney (1983) and many recent publications (e.g. Kershaw & Salvage 1986, Pearson & Vaughan 1986) could never be accused of using alienating language.

Nursing has been described as both an art and a science, but there are risks in accepting a strictly scientific approach and only those facts that can be tested or proved. Patients are far more than activities of living, systems, flexible lines of defence or stress adapters. Such approaches, if interpreted in a reductionist way, run contrary to the need to see the patient as a whole person. Not all that is seen can easily be researched; much of what happens between nurse and patient is so delicate and qualitative that it is difficult, if not impossible, to research it. While nurses should research and test most of what they do, they must never be afraid to accept the transient, unprovable, subjective and existential nature of their work.

Nursing's complexity leads to a tendency to emphasise the scientific, the technical and the observable as valuable and of higher status, but Lenara (1983) notes that the qualitative, living relationship is valuable in its own right. 'Basic' or 'menial' nursing is as valid and valuable as the 'high-tech' approach; favouring high-tech at the expense of high-touch leads nurses to see themselves in the 'narcissistic mirror offered by medicine' (Oakley 1984). Basic nursing is the essence of nursing – the skills required are complex, intricate and important in their own right. The heart of nursing is being with, helping, teaching; attending to the most fundamental of human needs. Lenara refers to them as heroic and argues that heroism is not confined to the battlefield or dramatic success over insuperable odds. A quieter, more subtle form of heroism marked by commitment to others is present in nursing. She writes: 'In nursing there are no small and useless tasks. Every little thing counts and every moment weighs, since each is offered for the welfare of human beings. The nurse's work is a composite of significant moments. The high degree of responsibility, the intensity of attention, the alertness of the continuous watching of the critically ill patient, the unpredictability of emergencies, the feverish and laborious task; these are neither exceptions nor recurring cycles. They formulate the everyday rule of the nurse's load. But above and beyond the intensive stress which characterises every single nursing moment, what is unknown and incomprehensible to many is the heroism of the nurse's heart which day by day, night by night, creates unique meanings of nursing. Nursing constitutes an everyday synthesis of all the elements in spiritual grandeur, a grandeur which is inseparable from life's tragedy. Pain and suffering, the tragic element of human life in its greatest intensity and sharpness, constitute the matrix of nursing. And this cannot be transcended without heroism.'

The thinking doer

Nursing, then, is doing – but nurses need to think too. A model should guide and direct nurses to produce 'thinking doers' – questioning, creative practitioners who have the problem-solving skills to deal with complex situations in a volatile and largely unpredictable setting.

No one model has all the answers, and nurses need to have a variety of them at their psychological fingertips. Many models focus on nurse and patient, yet ignore the complex influences of the outer world; in such a complex world, models can never be more than guidelines, collections of ideas, or gatherings of concepts to help with the job. They can never contain all that nursing is (as some theorists claim for their models) or can be; to suggest otherwise is pretentious and arrogant.

Models must liberate nurses, not enslave them. They should be launching platforms to creativity, not boxes in which nurses must confine their activities or their thoughts. Should nursing put itself into such a box, it may wake up to find that what it has really built for itself is a coffin. Models can help us, but they are not panaceas. Despite the many valid concerns and reservations, we need models – used creatively and critically – to be effective nurses.

References

Chenitz C & Swanson J (1985) *From Practice to Grounded Theory.* New York: Addison Wesley.

Dylak P (1986) The state of the art. *Nursing Times,* **82**(42), 72.

Graham C (1987) Front line revolt. *Nursing Times,* 22 April, 60.

Johnson M (1985) Model of perfection. *Nursing Times,* **82**(6), 42–44.

Kershaw B & Salvage J, eds (1986) *Models for Nursing.* Chichester: John Wiley.

Lenara V (1983) *Heroism as a Nursing Value.* Athens: The Sisterhood Evniki.

Lister P (1987) The misunderstood model. *Nursing Times,* **83**(41), 40–42.

Luker K (1988) Do models work? *Nursing Times,* **84**(5), 27–29.

Martin J (1984) *Hospitals in Trouble.* Oxford: Blackwell.

Menzies I (1961) A case study in the functioning of social systems as a defence against anxiety. *Human Relations,* **13,** 95–121.

Miller A (1985) Theories in nursing. *Nursing Times,* **8**(10), 14.

Nursing Standard (1987) Nurses are wonderful. *Nursing Standard,* **2**(7), 12.

Oakley A (1984) The importance of being a nurse. *Nursing Times,* **80**(50), 24–27.

Ottaway R (1976) A change strategy to implement new norms, new style and new environment in the work organisation. *Personnel Review,* **5**(1), 13–20.

Pearson A & Vaughan B (1986) *Nursing Models for Practice.* London: Heinemann.

Purdy E, Wright S & Johnson M (1988a) On the right track. *Nursing Times,* **84**(34), 44–45.

Purdy E, Wright S & Johnson M (1988b) Change for the better. *Nursing Times,* **84**(38), 34–36.

Reilly D (1975) Why a conceptual framework? *Nursing Outlook,* **23**(9), 566–599.

Roper N, Logan W & Tierney A (1983) *Using a Model for Nursing.* Edinburgh: Churchill Livingstone.

Sternberg P (1986) Models and theories have not changed practice. *Nursing Times,* 12 November, 12.

Webb C (1984) On the eighth day God created the nursing process and nobody rested. *Senior Nurse,* **1**(32), 22–25.

Wright S (1986) *Building and Using a Model of Nursing.* London: Edward Arnold.

Wright S (1988) Developing nursing: The contribution to quality. *International Journal of Health Care and Quality Assurance,* **1**(1), 12–15.

Models for Nursing 2
Edited by B Kershaw and J Salvage
© 1990 Scutari Press

4

Nursing Models and their Relationship to the Nursing Process and Nursing Theory

HELEN CHALMERS

Particular interest has focused on the development and potential usefulness of nursing models in the UK during the 1980s. Uncertainty has surrounded the differences, similarities and relationships between nursing theory, nursing models and the nursing process. In this chapter the nursing process will be briefly described and its limited value as a basis for informing nursing practice will be examined. The need for a knowledge base to underpin the use of the nursing process will be discussed, and the contribution that nursing models can make towards this will be explored. Finally, some differences between nursing models and nursing theory will be highlighted.

Historically, according to Johnson (1974), nursing has been regarded as an occupation requiring only physical strength and a degree of compassion to be effective. She argues that this has led to a denial of the intellectual nature of nursing and has hindered the development of a body of knowledge on which to base nursing practice: 'Nursing stands today as a field of practice without a scientific heritage – an occupation created by society long ago to offer a distinctive service, but one still ill defined in practical terms, a profession without the theoretical base it seems to require' (p.373).

The recent upsurge of interest in using nursing models as a possible means of informing what nurses do points to a greater acknowledgement of the intellectual nature of nursing. One reason for this may be nurses' growing desire to establish more firmly a recognised role in health care that goes beyond assisting doctors. Central to such a concern is a desire to provide high quality nursing care based on an identified body of nursing knowledge. Practising nurses who share this aim have been unable to ignore the emergence of nursing models, because they offer one way of informing what nurses do that may allow a higher standard of care.

Nurses seeking greater role clarification and a more reliable means of delivering a high standard of care have tended to become more questioning of what they do, why they do it and how well they do it. For many, the difficulty in finding satisfactory answers to such questions has further highlighted the lack of a theoretical basis for nursing practice.

This increased willingness to adopt a questioning approach may have led to the welcome given by some British nurses to the nursing process, following the publication of Yura and Walsh's well-known book, *The Nursing Process,* in 1967. Although some felt that the nursing process offered nothing new and some were openly concerned at the emphasis on documentation that quickly emerged, others felt that its systematic approach to what nurses do might help to answer some of the pressing questions being raised about the unique role of the nurse. In the early 1970s such questions were of concern not only to practising nurses but increasingly to other managers of health care resources, many of whom were non-nurses.

A more detailed consideration of what the nursing process is may help to clarify why, in itself, the nursing process has been largely inadequate to answer these questions.

The nursing process considered

Stevens (1984) has recently argued that three kinds of change can take place in nursing: those associated with the nursing act, those associated with the patient, and those associated with the interaction between the two. The nursing process focuses on the first of these positions in that it is primarily concerned with what nurses do. However, the way that a nurse carries out the nursing process will depend on many factors, some of which will relate to the patient and some to the rapport established between nurse and patient.

The nursing process divides what nurses do into a number of clearly defined and named stages. Although differences exist in the literature, these stages are generally known as assessment, planning, implementation (or intervention) and evaluation. It is easy to consider these as peculiar to nursing, but for most of us life is a continuous round of decision-making which looks remarkably similar. In order to prepare a meal, for example, a number of factors will need to be *assessed* or taken into account. It is important to know how many people require food, their likes and dislikes, and how much time is available to get things ready. Once this information is to hand, it will be possible to *plan* what food to buy and organise a timetable for its preparation. Subsequently this plan will be *implemented* via a number of activities. The necessary provisions will be acquired and the chosen dishes prepared. If the meal is ready on time and everyone appears satisfied, the process may be *evaluated* as having been successful.

This four-stage process, therefore, is one with which we are probably all familiar. How then does it become specifically the *nursing* process? In part it may be considered the nursing process when the four steps are carried out by nurses in the course of their work with patients or clients. However, the nursing process is far from explicit in guiding nurses towards particular styles of assessment, planning, implementation and evaluation. This inadequacy will be further explored before examining how nursing models might provide some necessary guidance on these matters.

By itself the nursing process is far from adequate as a means of planning and delivering nursing care (Aggleton & Chalmers 1986). Although it may advocate data-gathering or assessment, it fails to clarify the ways in which data might be gathered. Similarly, it does not help nurses select what is necessary from the wealth of information available about a patient. For example, when assessing patients, should nurses use a detailed checklist with the opportunity to record some of a limited set of responses, or should they adopt an open, reflective approach in which the focus is on gaining an understanding of the patient's perception of what is happening?

There are important implications both for the quality of the data gathered and for the relationship likely to develop between patient and nurse when a choice of this nature is made. For some patients an in-depth, probing interview may be regarded as an invasion of privacy. On the other hand, tightly structured assessment schemes tend to yield superficial data that rarely present a picture of the individual as a unique person. They are therefore often inadequate as a basis from which to plan care.

If practising nurses recognise that some degree of balance between these two rather extreme positions is likely to be needed, has the introduction of the nursing process contributed to this recognition? This seems unlikely, given that the nursing process does not operate with any particular view of people except perhaps that human beings have the ability to solve problems. However, nurses working, for example, with an understanding of people that highlights their uniqueness and their right to make choices about the health care they receive may favour particular approaches to seeking information. They are more likely to engage in assessment in a way that demonstrates sensitivity to the variety of data-gathering methods available.

The nursing process follows assessment with a goal-setting and planning stage. Here also the way in which the person is conceptualised will influence what takes place. If the patient is regarded as a passive recipient of the nursing process, then the nurse is likely to set goals and make prescriptive plans on his behalf. It has been all too common at this stage of the nursing process for goals to be set in terms of what *nurses* should achieve. This deflects attention away from patients and focuses instead on nurses and what they are doing. Some nurses may have interpreted the thrust of the planning stage in this way because the nursing process offers no guidance about planning and goal-setting. It is insufficient, though, simply to exhort nurses to set goals. There must be an explicit philosophy based on an understanding of people to guide nurses in their identification and setting of goals, and to suggest what the aims of nursing care might be.

If nursing is seen as a way of helping individuals to achieve their potential for self-care (Orem 1985), then the goals set should reflect this. On the other hand, nursing that seeks to assist people in their efforts to adopt new roles (e.g. Riehl 1980) may well focus on goals of a rather different nature.

Nursing interventions, too, will vary according to the overall aim of care and its relationship to the understanding of people which the nurse and patient share.

Sometimes nurses may be actively involved in doing things for patients; at other times they may be supporting and encouraging patients as they learn new skills. This does not mean that people can only benefit from one type of nursing intervention. Rather it acknowledges the diversity of skills needed in nursing, and highlights the importance of nurses being able to make informed choices about how best to intervene. The nursing process alone fails to inform such choices.

Yura and Walsh (1988) still assert that the evaluation stage is the most neglected part of the nursing process 'because it has been perceived as the most difficult' (p.174). Here, too, encouraging nurses to evaluate care is not enough. How should this take place and should it focus on patient outcomes or the completion of nursing actions to specified standards? Without appropriate guidelines it is hardly surprising that evaluation remains somewhat neglected, or that it is perceived as difficult. There is an enormous need for nurses to develop reliable and valid measuring tools to assist both in initial data-gathering and in formative and summative evaluation.

So far it has been argued that the nursing process alone, whilst encouraging nurses to involve themselves in a systematic series of specified tasks, gives inadequate guidance as to how such tasks might be accomplished. In the absence of such information, even experienced nurses may be tempted to act on the basis of intuition or may carry out the stages of the nursing process around a set of concerns derived from the medical model (Aggleton & Chalmers 1986).

An over-emphasis on the nursing process as a paper exercise gives additional concern in some care settings. The completion of pages of documentation is seen of itself to equate with the successful introduction of the process. Far from being a formality, nursing process documentation has been identified by many nurses as a useful means of promoting continuity of care between different care environments. Wilding, Wells and Wilson (1988) are recent advocates of this in their work in a neonatal unit, where a nursing model 'suited to the family-centred philosophy of care in the unit' (p.38) is in use.

Nursing models: developing the knowledge base

The preceding section examined the stages of the nursing process and questioned their adequacy as a means of informing nursing practice. What is required is a guiding philosophy and knowledge base that can begin to answer some of the dilemmas raised by the nursing process, several of which have been outlined above.

Some time ago Johnson (1974) discussed the possible ways in which nurses might proceed in their development of a knowledge base for nursing. She put forward three options which still have credence today. One is a laissez-faire approach in which there is little focused or coordinated activity. In this kind of situation nursing knowledge is likely to develop haphazardly. Secondly, nursing could continue with its past allegiance to medicine but, as Johnson has emphasised, 'progress toward a theoretical body of *nursing knowledge* via this route is inconceivable to anyone who envisions a distinctive professional identity for nursing' (p.374).

The third option, and the one favoured by Johnson and other nurse theorists, begins from an acceptance that nursing has something special and unique to offer people. Such a view imposes 'a significant social responsibility' (p.375) on nurses and demands that they practise from a knowledge base, central to which should be an understanding of the person, and from which guidelines for practice (or ways of informing the nursing process) can be developed. Here, Johnson is advocating the development of nursing theory, the beginnings of which may be found in nursing models.

It may be useful to return to Stevens' (1984) view that major trends in nursing tend to align themselves to the nursing act, the patient or the interaction between the two. The nursing process focuses primarily on what nurses do and is therefore necessarily limited in terms of what it can achieve. Nursing models endeavour to address all three of these positions by providing guidelines for what nurses do that emanate from an understanding of the nature of people and acknowledge the importance of the relationship between this understanding and what nurses do.

The well-known definition of a nursing model offered by Riehl and Roy (1980) may appear daunting at first: '... a systematically constructed, scientifically based, and logically related set of concepts which identify the essential components of nursing practice together with the theoretical basis of these concepts and values required for their use by the practitioner' (p.6). However, it contains some essential points that can help to identify certain key elements found in most nursing models.

It has been suggested (Aggleton & Chalmers 1986) that models of nursing are likely to have something to say about seven aspects of patient care. Such a list

Table 4.1   The similarities between seven key elements of a nursing model and a well-known definition of a nursing model

Seven key elements of a nursing model (after Aggleton & Chalmers 1986)	Definition of a nursing model (Riehl & Roy 1980)
1 The nature of people	'. . . a systematically constructed, scientifically based, and logically related set of concepts . . .'
2 The causes of problems likely to require nursing intervention	
3 The nature of assessment	'. . . the essential components of nursing practice . . .'
4 The nature of planning and goal-setting	
5 The nature of intervention	
6 The nature of evaluation	
7 The role of the nurse	'. . . values required for their use by the practitioner . . .'

is helpful when trying to make sense of models of nursing and can provide a useful first step for comparing one with another. Table 4.1 (above) demonstrates the similarities between these seven elements and Riehl and Roy's definition.

Nursing models are usually based on a variety of understandings about people that come from a number of disciplines. A model develops when such understandings are carefully examined to see how they might apply to the nature and practice of nursing. Nurse theorists have turned in particular to the disciplines of psychology, physiology and sociology in order to formulate nursing models. Within a particular nursing model certain aspects of the nature of people are likely to be seen as more important than others. It is when these significant aspects of people are considered that the stages of the nursing process become more informed.

It is not the purpose of this chapter to give detailed examples of how specific nursing models might affect the way in which these stages of the nursing process are carried out. Such examples can be found elsewhere in the text. However, it may serve as an introduction to consider some of the ways in which assessment, planning, intervention and evaluation may take place when working with a nursing model of a particular type.

A number of authors share the notion that three main types of nursing model can be identified, namely developmental, systems and interactionist models (Riehl & Roy 1980, Fawcett 1984, McFarlane 1986). However, such a categorisation should not be taken to mean that the differences between nursing models are absolute (Aggleton & Chalmers 1987). Rather a particular model may seek to emphasise developmental theories, systems theory or interactionist theory in its understanding of the nature of people. Table 4.2 therefore identifies some of the concerns that may characterise the use of the nursing process with a certain type of nursing model.

Well-constructed nursing models should enable nurses to plan and deliver nursing care based not on intuition, nor on a medical model of care, but on a set of understandings about people that can begin to inform all the stages of the nursing process.

The beginnings of nursing theory

In what ways do nursing models and nursing theory differ? Exploration of the literature emphasises the importance that many writers have given to this question (Fawcett 1984, Meleis 1985, Torres 1985).

Just as nursing models tend to originate from existing theory within the disciplines of physiology, psychology and sociology, so nursing models themselves can be regarded as a very early stage in the development of *nursing* theory. It may also be useful to consider nursing theory as a generic term to describe statements about nursing that are variable in the extent to which they attempt to describe, explain or predict relationships between phenomena.

It is unlikely that any particular nursing model will become accepted in its current form as nursing theory. What is more likely is that certain elements within a nursing model (or models) will come to be regarded as more reliable in terms

Table 4.2   The nursing process used with different types of nursing model

Type of model	Assessment	Planning	Intervention	Evaluation
Developmental e.g. Peplau 1952	Likely to focus on a person's stage of development as compared with 'normal' development, and how current circumstances might be inhibiting growth or causing regression Likely to value assessment as an ongoing, developing process	Likely to specify outcomes that demonstrate the attainment of new developmental goals or the re-establishment of a developmental stage from which the individual has regressed	Required to restore developmental progress and maturation Likely to emphasise the educative and counselling role of the nurse	Will search for evidence of growth and maturation
Systems e.g. Johnson 1980, Roy 1980, Roper, Logan & Tierney 1985	Likely to focus on how well parts of a person are functioning and whether the parts are achieving an overall state of balance Likely to have a structured assessment format for gathering information about each part of the system	Likely to specify short-term outcomes in a number of parts, with long-term goals specifying a state of homeostasis or balance The setting of priorities will be particularly important as changes in one part will affect others	Required to achieve balance within and between parts of the system Likely to advocate a variety of nursing roles depending on the type of systems model, e.g. biological systems models suggest nursing of a physical nature	Will search for evidence of homeostasis, which may be biological, psychological and/or social
Interactionist e.g. Travelbee 1971, Riehl 1980	Likely to focus on the development of rapport between nurse and patient/client Likely to focus on current role(s) and patient/client's perception of situation	Likely to favour short-term goals which are sensitive to developing relationships Likely to specify new role behaviours, and to emphasise the importance of negotiation in the setting of goals	Required to enable the taking on of new roles Likely to involve both nurse and client in activities that help them to see the situation from the other's point of view	Will search for evidence of new role performances

of what they say about the nature of people and their likely responses to difficult situations.

This might take place if a specific concept is found by practising nurses to be especially significant when planning and delivering care. For example, in the nursing models proposed by Roy (1980) and King (1981) there is considerable emphasis on the concepts of self and body image. Roy in her adaptation model identifies four adaptive modes within people, one of which, the self-concept mode, is concerned with individuals' views about their personal and physical selves. King identifies six important concepts within the personal system of individuals, of which two are the concepts of self and body image.

Although the models of Roy and King differ in many respects, there is a similar emphasis on the importance to people of their self-image and the way this can be disturbed during times of personal crisis. Such a notion, that when experiencing a particular difficulty a person may develop a distorted self-image, might constitute a theoretical statement at the descriptive level. It should not be regarded as an explanatory statement because it does not attempt to explain *why* self-image is disturbed.

However, King (1981) offers one possible explanation. She particularly identifies loss of function as a cause of body image distortion and supports this from both her own nursing experience and that of others. If such a relationship between loss of function and distorted body image is repeatedly supported by practising nurses in a variety of clinical settings, explanatory statements may be developed.

The most powerful theory is that which predicts relationships between phenomena. There is little evidence to suggest that there yet exists predictive theory that can reliably indicate those people whose perception of self and body image will be profoundly affected by loss of function of some part of their body. Indeed, there is little nursing knowledge that can claim to reach the level of predictive theory. The extensive work on the effect of prolonged pressure on the skin and underlying tissues perhaps comes closest to such a claim.

Nursing models may provide the beginnings of nursing theory. However, their value to the practice of nursing is yet to be reliably established and their use and critical evaluation by nurses in a variety of practice settings is essential. A defined knowledge base for nursing should help to clarify the role of the nurse and provide a means of achieving high standards of care. The opportunity that nursing models offer for the development of a knowledge base must not be ignored.

References

Aggleton P & Chalmers H (1986) *Nursing Models and the Nursing Process*. London: Macmillan.

Aggleton P & Chalmers H (1987) Models of nursing, nursing practice and nurse education. *Journal of Advanced Nursing,* **12**(5), 573–581.

Fawcett J (1984) *Analysis and Evaluation of Conceptual Models of Nursing.* Philadelphia: Davis.

Johnson D (1974) Development of theory: a requisite for nursing as a primary health profession. *Nursing Research,* **23**(5), 372–377.

Johnson D (1980) The behavioural system model for nursing. In Riehl J & Roy C, eds, *Conceptual Models for Nursing Practice.* Norwalk, CT: Appleton Century Crofts.

King I (1981) *A Theory for Nursing.* Chichester: John Wiley.

McFarlane J (1986) The value of models for care. In Kershaw B & Salvage J, eds, *Models for Nursing.* Chichester: John Wiley.

Meleis A (1985) *Theoretical Nursing.* London: Lippincott.

Orem D (1985) *Nursing: Concepts of Practice.* New York: McGraw-Hill.

Peplau H (1952) *Interpersonal Relations in Nursing.* New York: Putnam.

Riehl J (1980) The Riehl interaction model. In Riehl J & Roy C, eds, *Conceptual Models for Nursing Practice.* Norwalk, CT: Appleton Century Crofts.

Riehl J & Roy C, eds (1980) *Conceptual Models for Nursing Practice.* Norwalk, CT: Appleton Century Crofts.

Roper N, Logan W & Tierney A (1985) *The Elements of Nursing.* Edinburgh: Churchill Livingstone.

Roy C (1980) The Roy adaptation model. In Riehl J & Roy C, eds, *Conceptual Models for Nursing Practice.* Norwalk CT: Appleton Century Crofts.

Stevens B (1984) *Nursing Theory: Analysis, Application, Evaluation.* Boston: Little, Brown and Company.

Torres G (1985) The place of concepts and theories within nursing. In George J, ed, *Nursing Theories.* Englewood Cliffs: Prentice Hall.

Travelbee J (1971) *Interpersonal Aspects of Nursing*. Philadelphia: Davis.

Wilding C, Wells M & Wilson J (1988) A model for family care. *Nursing Times,* **84**(15), 38, 40–41.

Yura H & Walsh M (1967) *The Nursing Process*. Norwalk CT: Appleton Century Crofts.

Yura H & Walsh M (1988) *The Nursing Process.* Norwalk CT: Appleton Century Crofts.

Models for Nursing 2
Edited by B Kershaw and J Salvage
© 1990 Scutari Press

5
From Model to Care Plan

MIKE WALSH

A model of nursing is of little value unless it can be translated into clinical practice, and unless it brings about an improvement in patient care. These two key issues will be tackled in this chapter.

Models of nursing are all based on the assumption that a patient-centred care approach is in use, and so the first step in translating a model into nursing practice is to be sure that the clinical area is fully conversant with the requirements of individualised patient care. Task allocation will undermine and destroy the whole philosophy of any nursing model. The phrase 'nursing process' is much misunderstood and has become a cliché, a scapegoat for those who resent change and wish to remain with their heads buried in the sands of nursing history. 'Individualised patient care' is a better and more accurate term, and will therefore be used throughout this chapter in describing the method used to plan and deliver care.

The next step is to consider the type of area in which the model is to be introduced. At this stage the nurse should think about what approach is most suitable for the patient's needs. She should beware the trap of working alone: discussions with patients and other members of the therapeutic team should allow the formulation of a broadly acceptable philosophy of care. It is then possible to consider various models and decide which one best reflects the agreed philosophy of care. The model must fit the patients, not vice versa. It may be confusing, however, to have several different models in any one setting; a unit should choose one model only: that which best fits its requirements. For example, a surgical unit may feel that an important aspect of recovery is successful adaptation to surgery, such as stoma formation, and may therefore choose the Roy adaptation model (Rambo 1984). Units specialising in trauma/accident and emergency or care of the elderly may consider the self-care aspect to be crucial and choose Orem's self-care model (Orem 1985, Walsh 1985). Staff caring for mentally ill people may decide that an interactionist approach is needed, and choose a model such as that of Riehl and Roy (1980).

It is doubtful whether models in their present stage of development can be applied across a health authority in blanket form. The diversity of patient conditions and needs is so great that it may never be possible to develop a 'general nursing model' that can be applied to any clinical situation. Authoritarian attempts by senior nurses to impose a single model show their lack of understanding of nursing models and good management in roughly equal proportions.

Armed with a suitable model and a commitment to individualised patient care, the nurse is now ready to translate theory into practice. This involves one of the hardest jobs of all, introducing change into nursing. Hunt (1987) and Alexander and Orton (1988) have shown that an individual nurse trying to bring about change has little chance of success: the inertia of the system is far too great. Successful change, as these researchers have shown, depends on a coordinated approach involving management, teachers and clinical staff working together on a project over a substantial period of time. The introduction of a nursing model requires this same integrated approach.

The need for effective assessment

If individualised patient care is to be practised, effective assessment is essential. There is no other way to discover a patient's individual problems. A garage mechanic will not try to repair a car without carrying out a detailed assessment to discover the cause of the problem, nor would a surgeon embark on an operation without similar investigation and assessment. Without a careful patient assessment, there can be no professional nursing care.

Filling in patient assessment forms on admission occupies a great many nursing hours, however, and the demands this makes on nursing time are often cited as one of the reasons why 'the nursing process doesn't work'. In day-to-day practice, a great deal of nursing time is undoubtedly wasted on assessment, because much of the information collected is irrelevant or is not used in nursing care. The problem tends to be compounded by the fact that much crucial information is missed altogether. Why should this be, and how can the use of a model help to avoid this problem?

The root of the problem lies in the documentation many nurses are forced to work with in trying to carry out planned, individualised care. Many poor quality assessment forms are not based on any rational model, so information is gathered in a disjointed way that is not related to the nursing care needed by the patient. The nurse feels obliged to fill in all the boxes, resulting in 30 minutes being spent admitting one patient, be he a fit young man having an ingrowing toenail removed under local anaesthetic or a middle-aged woman undergoing mastectomy for cancer. The focus of the assessment is not the patient, but the forms – all of which must be completed. Little is learned about the patient in such an assessment, and even less is actually used in planning care.

The use of a model of nursing changes this and makes assessment a meaningful and worthwhile use of nursing time, as the assessment procedure now has a rational structure. For example, if the philosophy is centred around self-care, an assessment may be carried out that focuses on the patient's self-care abilities in the manner suggested by Orem. Nursing staff need to study the model and design their own assessment form based on the philosophy of the model and best suited to their requirements.

The authors of the various models have offered their own assessment schemes. It is important that nurses do not see them simply as headings or a checklist of things to look at. They must assess what the model requires under each heading. Thus Roy's model requires an assessment of various areas of physiology, and headings such as nutrition and elimination are listed. This means more than measuring the patient's height and weight and asking how often he opens his bowels – such information could be sought using any philosophy. To practise the Roy model, the nurse needs to find out how the patient adapts to his height and weight, how it affects his life and, in the second-level assessment, what are the likely causes of obesity or whatever maladaptation is present. Similarly, how does the patient adapt to being constipated – is he taking laxatives bought at the chemist or some other home remedy? It is not enough to discover that the patient has problems with incontinence of urine. How does this affect his life, what measures does he take to cope with it – in other words, how is he adapting?

An assessment based on a model needs to be more than a checklist of items such as nutrition or elimination. It needs to incorporate the philosophy that drives the model; it needs to answer a number of questions, such as how the patient is achieving independence, practising self-care or adapting to the daily requirements of nutrition or elimination.

Nurses should also be encouraged to be realistic in the depth of their assessment, and assess only what is relevant to the patient's needs. A nursing assessment that takes three times as long as the surgery the patient is to undergo is not a very sensible use of time. The use of a model in care planning will use the nurse's time better by structuring the assessment process and ensuring that only relevant information is gathered.

Problems – from the patient's perspective

Having made an assessment that reflects the chosen model, the next step is to deduce from it the patient's problems. Common mistakes seen in care planning are problem statements that are too vague (such as 'risk of infection') or are not patient-centred. The problem must be stated precisely, and in terms that make it clear that it is the *patient's* problem. Failure to achieve this will contribute to goals that are inappropriate or unmeasurable. If the nurse is using a model to guide the care-planning exercise, patient problems must also be seen in the light of the model. Thus an immediate postoperative patient might be 'unable to maintain their own airway', a self-care deficit in Orem's model; a patient who has undergone stoma formation might be 'unable to look at stoma', a maladaptation in Roy's model.

Although jargon should not be used for the sake of it, the statements of patient problems should as far as possible reflect the language and philosophy of the model. If the language of the model is not used in stating patient problems, there is a serious risk that the rest of the care planning, and hence the care itself, will not reflect the model of choice. The model will be little more than window-dressing to impress the National Board inspector, similar to the way the nursing process is carried out in many wards today. When a model is chosen it must be more than a paper exercise or a checklist for assessment; it is a model of nursing that must be translated into the care the patient receives.

A feature of any one unit or ward is that many patients have common problems. This has led nurses to consider the amount of the time spent writing out care plans, which may be repetitive in that they document similar problems and asso-ciated care for many patients. If two patients are to have a cholecystectomy or a mastectomy, certain areas of preoperative and postoperative care are common to both types of surgery – although there are also major differences, not least of which the fact that the patients are two different people. The pressures of time and the identification of common problems has led to the development of common core care plans. This involves nurses discussing the problems most commonly found and drafting a plan to deal with them. Such plans can be preprinted ready for use with each patient as they are admitted. Examples are given by Walsh (1985) in accident and emergency; Glasper, Martin and Stonehouse (1987) in children's care; and Foster (1987) in intensive care.

The disadvantage of this approach is the risk that the patient is no longer seen as an individual, with care planning neglected in favour of a series of standar-dised problems that all patients are assumed to have. On the other hand, if the time saved by using the core care plan is used to look at the patient's individual problems, it could be a major aid to care and to teaching.

The development of core care plans also offers the innovative nurse a splendid opportunity in introducing a model of nursing to an area of care. In drafting the core plans, she can ensure that the model's approach is followed to problem formulation, goal-setting and hence to nursing care. The core care plans act as an example for nurses to follow in writing out the individualised sections of the care plans, helping to reinforce the model in use.

Formulation of core plans must be a collective exercise involving all trained staff on a unit, essential to ensure the highest quality plan and staff cooperation in its use. Nurses are more likely to use the model if they feel they contributed to the plan, and if they feel involved they are more likely to be committed to the success of the initiative.

Setting goals

After identifying the patient's problems, the next step is to set goals that are patient-centred, realistic and measurable. Great confusion arises because much of the documentation in use does not refer to goals but to aims. This begs the question, whose aims? The focus of care is the patient, so it is illogical to write nursing aims at the stage of care planning; yet it is common to find nursing aims written here, and not patient goals. If the nurse is using a rational, patient-centred model of nursing the requirement at this stage is for clearly stated patient goals. 'Patient will not develop pressure sores' is a patient goal; to write 'Prevent pressure sores' makes a statement of nursing care, but it is not a patient goal. This confusion arises partly because of the poor design of much of the documentation, and a lack of understanding of what individualised care is trying to achieve. A column headed 'Aims' is hopelessly vague, as it fails to make clear whose aims we are talking about. 'Patient goals' would be a more correct and unambiguous heading.

Nurses and doctors have traditionally exercised tight control over patients; nurses automatically start writing about nursing aims, and fail to see the individual patient as the focus of care. In using a model the nurse must accept that one of the things it is trying to achieve is to shift the focus to the individual patient; nursing must now start to look at patient goals as the hub of care, and reflect this in care planning.

The goals set should reflect the philosophy of the model, so they should be couched in terms of achieving independence, self-care, adaptation and so on. They should also be realistic and measurable. It is not realistic to state that an elderly patient will achieve independence in dressing within two weeks if he has just had a major cerebrovascular accident leaving him with a severe hemiplegia.

Experience has shown that care plans abound with statements such as 'correct dehydration'; the old chestnut 'push fluids' is still alive and well. First, these are statements about nursing aims or actions, not patient goals, and secondly, they are unmeasurable. How does the nurse know when dehydration has been corrected? What criteria are used to measure success or failure? If the goal is stated as 'patient to consume 2.5 litres fluids by 9 p.m.', that can be measured.

Goals must therefore be patient-centred and realistic, and reflect the philosophy of the model, written in a way that is measurable. To write 'Patient will achieve self-care in dressing by 1.10.88' appears to meet those criteria, but does it? What is meant by self-care in the Orem model? It could mean that the patient will dress himself with no assistance, or with some assistance; either way he has overcome his self-care deficit and got dressed. Furthermore, how long has it taken him to dress and is this an acceptable time? Confusion could easily arise if Nurse A expects the patient to dress unaided by 10 a.m. but the following day Nurse B interprets this to mean that as long as she helps the patient with his shoes and socks and the patient does the rest by 11 a.m. all is well. Despite one statement of a patient goal, different nurses are moving the goalposts every day! Goal-setting therefore needs to be precise. Just as in a race the competitors need to know where the finishing line is, so in nursing the patient and nurse need to know exactly what goal they are striving for.

Achievement of a goal is more likely if the nurse and patient have agreed on it. Patient involvement in goal-setting and care planning is greatly to be desired. Some models, such as Riehl's interactionist approach (Riehl and Roy 1980), stress the importance of the patient's perspective, but other theorists have been weak in appreciating this crucial dimension. In using a model, the nurse must always involve the patient and try to see things from his point of view.

The effects on nursing practice

Will the use of a model actually change nursing in practice? What are the effects on nursing interventions of using model A compared with model B? If the answer is none, there does not seem to be a lot of point in trying to use the model. The use of a model's assessment scheme and some slight changes in the headings on the care plan are not sufficient to justify the statement that the ward has introduced that model. The model's philosophy must be reflected in the care carried out – the nursing interventions practised. For example, if Orem is used, is the traditional drug round justified? If patients are to learn to be self-caring, they should be taught about their medication and enabled to practise self-care by being responsible under supervision for their own medication while on the ward. Or consider a 45-year-old woman who is to undergo mastectomy; she must adapt postoperatively to having one breast. The nurse using Roy should therefore plan ways of helping her adapt, from encouraging her to express her feelings, and giving practical hints, through to talking to her sexual partner.

The introduction of a model should start to raise questions about a great deal of ritualistic nursing practice. A new model brings new approaches to nursing, and changes in traditional practice. Nursing cannot carry on as before. The practitioners will have to explain the changes not only to their peers, but also to other staff and to the patients. Discussions are essential with staff such as doctors, physiotherapists and occupational therapists. The philosophy behind the care should be explained to the patient and family; otherwise there may be major misunderstandings. Effective patient care requires teamwork, and the introduction of a model is no exception.

The introduction of a model to care planning should be tackled carefully, as such a major step has many ramifications and implications. Whatever model is chosen, its main aim will be individualised patient care. To succeed, the nursing should be organised using a method known as primary nursing. This concept involves one nurse being responsible for a patient's care 24 hours a day, even when she is off duty (Wright 1987, MacGuire 1988). This can be done effectively only by care planning which permits the nurse allocated to the patient to see what is required simply from looking at the care plan. The team nursing system commonly used today contributes to the failure of care planning, as no one nurse is ever responsible for one patient's care. Every few hours there is a complete change of personnel, while we hear 'We don't do the nursing process at night or in the evening' (or at weekends or in the afternoon?).

The final question is how to evaluate the effectiveness of change. Accurate tools are needed to measure the quality of care both before and after the introduction of an individualised system of care based on a nursing model. Simply asking patients if they were satisfied with their care is not good enough. Much more sensitive and reliable tools are needed to determine whether standards of care have been improved as a result of introducing a model. Much work is now going on to develop quality assurance in nursing; the results will be invaluable in assessing the effectiveness of models in practice. If it cannot be demonstrated that a model improves patient care, of what value is that model to clinical nurses?

References

Alexander M & Orton H (1988) Research in action. *Nursing Times,* **84**(8), 38–41.
Foster D (1987) The development of care plans for the critically ill patient. *Nursing,* **3**(15), 571–573.

Glasper A, Martin L & Stonehouse J (1987) Core care plans. *Nursing Times,* **83**(10), 55–57.

Hunt M (1987) The process of translating research findings into nursing practice. *Journal of Advanced Nursing,* **12**(1), 101–110.

MacGuire J (1988) I'm your nurse. *Nursing Times*, **84**(30), 32–36.

Orem D (1985) *Nursing: Concepts of Practice.* New York: McGraw-Hill.

Rambo B (1984) *Adaptation Nursing.* New York: Saunders.

Riehl J & Roy C, eds, (1980) *Conceptual Models for Nursing Practice.* Norwalk, CT: Appleton Century Crofts.

Walsh M (1985) *Accident and Emergency Nursing: A New Approach.* London: Heinemann.

Wright S (1987) Patient-centred practice. *Nursing Times,* **83**(38), 24–27.

Models for Nursing 2
Edited by B Kershaw and J Salvage
© 1990 Scutari Press

6

Patient Education: A Model Approach

DIANA CARTER

This chapter aims to discuss the application of the Riehl interaction model in the context of patient education. It does not go into detail about the process of patient education; this information can be found in more specialised texts (e.g. DuBrey 1982, Narrow 1979, Redman 1984). The use of nursing models in patient education is an area of nursing care that has not been adequately researched, and many of the ideas in this chapter form part of a research project that has not yet been completed.

The terms 'patient teaching' and 'patient education' are used interchangeably throughout, although, as Simonds (1979) explains, 'teaching' refers to only one component of the patient education process, namely the imparting of information. 'Patient education' is the process of influencing patient behaviour, producing changes in knowledge, attitudes and skills required to maintain and improve health.

Patient education is an essential aspect of total patient care, as emphasised by Sechrist (1979), who pointed out that patients require information about their health care in order to assist them to return to a previous state of wellness and/or to prevent the occurrence or recurrence of illness states. More recently, Price (1984) stated that it is the central component of the rehabilitation process. Yet studies carried out in the 1960s were among the first to draw attention to a failure on the part of health care personnel to meet patients' teaching needs. Patients thought the information they received in hospital was insufficient, contradictory and confusing (Cartwright 1964, Duff & Hollingshead 1968).

Individual needs for patient education

Efforts must be maximised to ensure that the information presented to patients is individualised and understandable. It is also important to recognise that it must be considered useful by the patient if he is to attend to and comprehend the teaching carried out by nurses. The desire for information forms a potent variable in determining what information a person receives and how it is interpreted. As Dodge (1969) has pointed out, understanding is facilitated when the person receives the kind of information he feels he needs in a particular situation. For most people illness and hospitalisation represent conditions of stress, and Dodge recognised that expressed cognitive needs might be at variance with what objective reality demands. Other writers have highlighted discrepancies between nurses' and patients' perceptions of learning needs (Lauer, Murphy & Powers 1982; Tilley, Gregor & Thiessen 1987).

An aspect of patient knowledge specific to each individual was put forward by Taylor (1965), who identified three temporal focuses affecting a person's need to know. A past focus searches to understand the cause of his present situation, reflecting a need to 'appease his gods' and relieve feelings of guilt. A present focus reflects a need to achieve immediate relief from symptoms and anxieties through immediate gratification. A future focus wrestles with long-term implications, and the paramount need is to plan or work towards the future. Taylor underlines the need for an individual educational diagnosis by stating that patients with different temporal focuses may need different items of information under apparently similar conditions, and will use the same items of information in different ways and for different purposes.

Averill (1973) says people seek to employ three different types of control over their lives – behavioural, decisional and cognitive; Price (1984) suggests that rather than being diminished during illness, the attempt to control events is increased as most people resent being dependent on others. Behavioural control is an attempt to manage overtly the events affecting the individual, and implies active measures being openly employed to modify circumstances. Decisional control is the attempt to set an order to events, implying the option of choices such as the decision to take one course of action rather than another. Cognitive control involves the ability to create an overall mental image of one's circumstances, and implies an understanding of the likely sequence of events and how such events are likely in turn to modify feelings and status. If patient education is combined in all three areas of control, the patient will be provided with a balanced understanding of what is happening, and will thereby be motivated to learn. Controlling any altered circumstances imposed by the illness and/or treatment should enable the patient to leave hospital sooner, reduce the need for repeated admission, and encourage continuing independence.

Independence – the ability to live life in a full and individual way without excessive support from others – calls for the exercise of control over any altered circumstances such as those resulting from illness. It is thus an essential component of the three major categories of goals or purposes of patient education that Narrow (1979) has identified (Table 6.1). By including within the process of patient education the means to enable the patient to know (Taylor 1965) and to control altered circumstances (Averill 1973), the individual can be helped in his struggle for independence (Figure 6.1).

The traditional approach to patient education from the perspective of the medical model highlights diagnosis, prognosis and therapy, with teaching

Table 6.1   Categories of purposes of patient education (Narrow 1979)

Category	Purposes
1 Teaching to promote health	Teaching that helps to improve quality of life, facilitate optimal physical and psychological growth and development, enhance self-esteem and promote self-actualisation
2 Teaching to prevent illness	Teaching directed towards assisting to eliminate or reduce the incidence of preventable illness and disease
3 Teaching to cope with illness	Teaching that grasps the notion that the patient and his family need to learn how to participate in the prescribed nursing and medical regimens, and how to live with a condition that cannot be cured or relieved.

oriented towards imparting knowledge about these three areas. This has largely been replaced by a more holistic approach in which the person is viewed as a total, non-fragmented human being who is the sum of all his parts. Instead of the nurse being interested solely in the diseased or dysfunctional part, concern is for the total person. It follows that patient education should include much more than teaching about a single, dysfunctional problem.

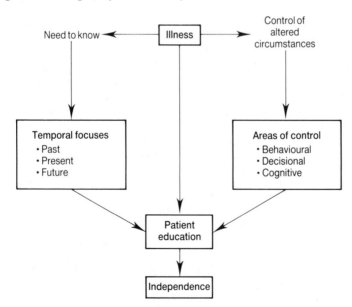

Figure 6.1   The process of patient education

This holistic concept of the human being, coupled with the move towards individualised, goal-directed nursing care through a process approach, provides the opportunity to consider patient education in care planning to achieve any or all of the broad goals outlined above. Indeed, it is virtually impossible not to use some form of process approach in professional practice; this suggested approach to patient education follows a parallel course to the nursing process. Patient education, however, is not a separate entity divorced from the other components of patient care. It should be seen as an integrated part of the nursing care process, with the patient, family and significant others fully involved at all stages.

Riehl's interaction model

How can the use of a nursing model contribute to patient education? For reasons which will later become clear, I have chosen Riehl's interaction model. This is an interesting model, which has been developed from symbolic interaction theory. Riehl argues that people constantly strive to make sense of the environments in which they find themselves. Additionally, everyone is said to differ in how he makes sense of a particular situation; when faced with the unfamiliar, he will tend to draw on past experience (Riehl 1980).

Symbolic interactionists describe social situations as being negotiated. Any definition of what a particular situation is about therefore arises out of interactions between all those present, in which different versions of the same reality come to be tested against one another. Take, for example, a patient who, two days after surgery to remove varicose veins, insists on remaining in bed and refuses to participate in any way in meeting his hygiene needs. The nurse, aware of the disadvantages and possible dangers of prolonged inactivity, is likely to want the patient to modify his attitudes and behaviour. The respective versions of reality are in conflict. The patient may regard the physical discomforts and the fact that he had an operation only two days ago as justification for remaining in bed (and attempting to claim the privileges of the sick role). Renegotiation is called for – between patient and nurse – of a social reality that is mutually acceptable.

Riehl sees three major systems or parameters as affecting a person's behaviour – physiological, psychological and sociological. Problems can arise when there are disturbances within one or more of these parameters, and an interrelationship between parameters is also recognised, disturbance of one possibly affecting the functioning of another. For example, the person with bronchial asthma who is extremely anxious, upset or excited about something (psychological parameter) may subsequently experience an acute attack of bronchospasm (physiological parameter). Depending on the nature of the factor that initially caused him to be anxious, upset or excited he may, in future, have to modify his social behaviour (sociological parameter) to avoid similar provocation.

Although other models may stress the importance of the physiological, the Riehl model pays particular attention to the importance of the psychological and sociological parameters as the critical systems affecting behaviour.

As Abbey (1980) points out, a person normally assumes responsibility for controlling particular factors such as nutrition and communication (Table 6.2), but

Table 6.2   Abbey's FANCAP factor as a basis for patient assessment (Abbey 1980)

F	Fluids
A	Aeration
N	Nutrition
C	Communication
A	Activity
P	Pain

surrenders this control in varying degrees during illness. Patient education can make a valuable contribution towards the individual's endeavours to regain control and independence in these activities of living, and Abbey's FANCAP mnemonic offers a systematic basis for the initial assessment of the patient.

Riehl explains that the nurse attempts to gain insight into the patient's subjective perception of his problems, and to ascertain the roles he has previously adopted to cope with similar problems. In other words, she tries to acquire an 'intersubjective understanding' of the ways the patient perceives the situation, and to assess the range of role performance open to him to help him to cope. This is said to help determine the degree of flexibility open to the patient, and also anticipate problems that might arise when the nurse encourages him to develop a new role in order to cope with a particular problem associated with his present or future health status.

A teaching strategy that can be employed to advantage in the context of this interaction model and patient education is that of *exploration*. The basis of exploration is that answers to problems come from the patient himself – the solutions lie within the person who is experiencing the problem or difficulty. It involves:

● helping the patient to examine the situation and/or his feelings about it;
● helping the patient to identify possible responses or courses of action;
● helping the patient to consider the likely consequences of the possible responses or courses of action available.

The patient may require more information about his illness and/or treatment in order fully to consider his feelings, courses of action and so on, but exploration *per se* should help develop role flexibility, and also give the nurse an understanding of the patient's view of the situation.

Exploration calls for an intense application of basic communcation skills. The nurse has to listen carefully, encourage the patient to express his feelings, help him to examine all possible aspects of the situation, use questions judiciously, clarify her own perceptions of the situation and share them with him, and help him to discover relationships between ideas and values. She must also convey empathy and concern, and refrain from giving advice or additional information until a desired behavioural course of action is chosen by the patient and/or specific help is requested (Narrow 1979).

Nurses sometimes have a tendency to identify problems *for* patients, to offer unsolicited advice and to tell the patient what he should or should not do. Clearly the Riehl interaction model calls for a different approach; one which is patient-centred. Exploration is a technique that will help us to apply the principles inherent in Riehl's model, and it also incorporates recognition of Taylor's temporal focuses and Averill's types of control. Additional information, new skills and so on can be incorporated as appropriate to help the patient adopt the new role he has chosen as a means of coping with his health-related problems (Figure 6.2).

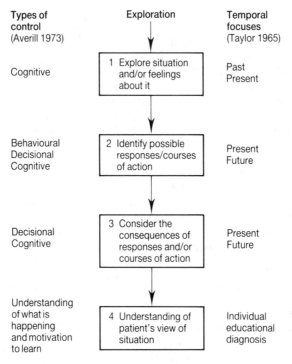

Figure 6.2   Patient education incorporating exploration in conjunction with types of control and temporal focuses

Case study

Mr Morris, a 45-year-old double-glazing salesman, has been admitted for investigation of recurrent attacks of chest pain said to be associated with physical exertion. Investigations reveal an elevated serum cholesterol level and areas of narrowing in the coronary arteries. A medical diagnosis of angina pectoris is made.

Using the FANCAP categories of assessment, areas of teaching need can be identified. A challenging aspect of patient education in this case involves helping Mr Morris to control his pain through the identification of those life events that are found to precipitate anginal attacks. The pain is reported to occur in conjunction with physical exertion, but further assessment and exploration helps the patient and the nurse to see that emotionally stressful situations also tend to precipitate the attacks. Thus it would appear that the physiological, psychological and sociological parameters referred to by Riehl are implicated. Through exploration the nurse can help Mr Morris to re-evaluate his lifestyle:

1   To reflect on the areas of his life that are physically and emotionally stressful to the extent that they cause him to experience chest pain.

2   To reflect on those areas which, through modification, may lead to a reduction in physical and emotional stress – thereby decreasing the incidence of chest pain.

3   To reflect on how such modifications could be achieved, i.e. the development of role flexibility.

In this way the nurse will acquire what Riehl calls an intersubjective understanding of the patient's perception of the problem and possible ways in which he can overcome it.

Mr Morris may require additional information to help him understand the situation fully. For example, he may need a simple explanation of the coronary blood supply, the pathological changes that have occurred in his coronary arteries, the physiological effects of exercise on the heart, and the implications of the pathological changes that have been found in his coronary arteries.

Exploration may show that Mr Morris has little difficulty understanding the link between physical stress and anginal pain, but is somewhat bewildered as to why emotional stress can also cause him to experience pain. Again, the nurse can provide information to facilitate this understanding, thus helping Mr Morris to appreciate that avoidance of particular social situations and/or alternative ways of dealing with them (role flexibility) will reduce the likelihood of further pain attacks. She will also need to explain about the prophylactic and therapeutic use of any prescribed medication. The use of role play could help Mr Morris to see that he can effectively prevent and/or treat anginal attacks in the future (Figure 6.3).

The initial assessment, subsequent exploration and identification of any additional information required by the patient are sources of goals or educational objectives. As the interaction between patient and nurse proceeds, these goals will hopefully be achieved. As part of the process (and contributing to the ongoing evaluation of the patient's progress towards the goals/educational objectives), the nurse will also be extending the accuracy of her subjective understanding of the patient's needs. Additionally, as the patient is encouraged to consider all aspects of the situation, he will be more able to develop the role flexibility required to help him cope in future and thereby maintain his independence.

Conclusion

This case study has considered only one aspect of the patient's learning needs – pain control – but it has hopefully served to illustrate the application of the principles inherent in Riehl's interaction model.

Patient's name: Mr. William Morris   Ward: 24   Date: 10.9.88

Category of assessment	Problem	Exploration	Additional information required	Teaching aids/ activities to assist
PAIN	Chest pain in relation to: (a) physical exertion (b) emotional stress	1 Explore feelings and situation Can identify activities which result in pain, but doesn't fully understand link. No understanding of link between emotion and pain, but can identify situations which give rise to pain.	Explain blood supply to myocardium; pathological changes, possible causes. Physiological effects of stress; implications in light of pathological changes in arteries.	Diagrams – heart and coronary circulation; normal and arteriosclerotic arteries.
		2 Responses/courses of action Has identified physical activities which can be reduced. Needs to learn how to resist/ avoid 'rising to the bait'. Self-administration of medication as prescribed.	Suggest possible ways of responding to provocations. Correct administration of drugs.	Role play Demonstration. Role play.
		3 Consequences of responses/courses of action May be times when it is impossible to avoid pain-inducing stress. Will try to take medication prophylactically. Therapeutic drug administration should not present any problems.		

Figure 6.3   Care plan for Mr Morris

Using exploration and providing additional information as required will have contributed towards satisfying the patient's temporal focuses affecting his need to know (Taylor 1965). Why the condition has occurred (past focus), how the symptoms can be relieved (present focus), and the long-term implications (future focus) have all been considered.

The patient has also been given the opportunity to employ the different types of control put forward by Averill (1973). For example, alternative ways of coping with potentially stressful situations (behavioural control) are now available to him. The information provided in relation to normal physiology and pathological changes contributes to cognitive control. Decisional control has been facilitated in that now, on the basis of his learning, he has the option of deciding on a particular course of action to help to prevent and/or control his chest pain.

Some of these ideas are still, admittedly, tentative. However, the use of a model-based approach to patient education is an area of nursing that merits urgent research.

References

Abbey J (1980) FANCAP: what is it? In Riehl J & Roy C, eds, *Conceptual Models for Nursing Practice*. Norwalk, CT: Appleton Century Crofts.

Averill J (1973) Personal control over aversive stimuli and its relationship to stress. *Psychological Bulletin,* **80,** 286–303.

Cartwright A (1964) *Human Relations and Hospital Care.* London: Routledge and Kegan Paul.

Dodge J (1969) Factors related to patients' perceptions of their cognitive needs. *Nursing Research,* **18**(6), 502–513.

DuBrey R (1982) *Promoting Wellness in Nursing Practice.* St Louis: CV Mosby Co.

Duff R & Hollingshead A (1968) *Sickness and Society.* New York: Harper and Row.

Lauer P, Murphy S & Powers M (1982) Learning needs of cancer patients: a comparison of nurse and patient perceptions. *Nursing Research,* **31**(1), 11–16.

Narrow B (1979) *Patient Teaching in Nursing Practice.* New York: John Wiley.

Price B (1984) A framework for patient education. *Nursing Times,* **80**(32), 28–30.

Redman B (1984) *The Process of Patient Education.* St Louis: Toronto.

Riehl J (1980) The Riehl interaction model. In Riehl J & Roy C, eds, *Conceptual Models for Nursing Practice.* Norwalk, CT: Appleton Century Crofts.

Sechrist K (1979) The effect of repetitive teaching on patients' knowledge about drugs to be taken at home. *International Journal of Nursing Studies,* **16,** 51–58.

Simonds S (1979) *National Task Force on Training Family Physicians in Patient Education: a Handbook for Teachers.* Philadelphia: Lippincott.

Taylor C (1965) The hopitalised patient's social dilemma. *American Journal of Nursing,* **65,** 96–99.

Tilley J, Gregor F & Thiessen V (1987) The nurse's role in patient education: incongruent perceptions among nurses and patients. *Journal of Advanced Nursing,* **12,** 291–301.

Models for Nursing 2
Edited by B Kershaw and J Salvage
© 1990 Scutari Press

7

Models and Midwifery

CHRISTINE HENDERSON

This chapter will seek to do four things:

- explore the reasons for a rejection of nursing models by some midwives;
- discuss the extent of their use in midwifery practice;
- describe the development of a model for midwifery;
- illustrate its use in practice.

The relevance of nursing models and the nursing process to midwifery practice provokes speculation. Confusion still exists between the terms 'process' and 'models', and their relevance to nursing continues to be questioned. British nurses were expected to introduce the nursing process in the late 1970s, as directed by the General Nursing Council for England and Wales (GNC 1977), but tutors and service nurses had little understanding of its underlying philosophy (Nursing Education Research Unit 1986). This resulted in resentment and rejection by many, a situation still found in some health authorities today. The use of the nursing process alone as a framework for practice is criticised by many as an 'empty approach' (a view supported by Aggleton & Chalmers 1986).

Exhorting nurses to carry out the nursing process without a chosen model of nursing as a framework is of little value. It is like constructing a building without the architect's plan. Unfortunately the nursing process was introduced before nursing models, leading to a failure to understand that the nursing process is not in itself a model of nursing, but rather a systematic approach to care. A model is the framework on which to base practice; the process is the means by which it is implemented.

Clifford (1988) points out that the question of the 1970s was 'Are you using the nursing process?' but in the 1980s it was 'Which model of nursing are you using?' – which added to the confusion and created divisions between theory and practice. The same confusion exists in midwifery, with few institutions recognising the relevance of models of nursing to midwifery practice. Evidence received by the Nursing Process Working Group indicated that a few midwifery units were trying to introduce the process, but the comments of the Royal College of Midwives reflect the views of many midwives: 'the problem-solving approach of the nursing process was more suited to a sickness model of care and ... as the care of the mother and baby did not belong to any one group of carers, the application of a process based on the contribution of one group was not appropriate ...' (Nursing Education Research Unit 1986).

One of the reasons why midwives reject nursing models and the nursing process relates to how they view midwifery and their role, i.e. as different from nursing – a point of contention among both groups which creates attitudinal problems. A resumé of the origins of the two professions may serve to highlight the reasons for this rejection.

Midwifery and nursing: separate development

Historically nursing and midwifery have developed separately. Nursing, with a concern for caring for the sick mainly in a hospital setting, was granted registration in 1919 but the GNC was not charged with the 'responsibility or resources to organise nurse education' nor with controlling the practice of nurses, but purely with maintaining a register (Davies 1980). Midwifery has a 'long genealogy' and was one of the few female occupations which had formal, recognised public status in the premedical era (Versluysen 1980). Registration was granted in 1902, and the Central Midwives Board was given the responsibility of supervising the practice and determining the training needs of midwives.

The midwife supported the mother in the process of childbirth, with the mother and baby normally in a state of health; until the late 1930s childbirth was an event usually occurring in the home. However pressure from medical bodies and successive governments succeeded in changing the place of childbirth and led to a different perception of midwifery and the role of the midwife: the mother was now viewed as a patient, and the adoption of a 'sick role model' was criticised in numerous reports on the maternity services. With the change in the place of birth, midwifery and midwife became synonymous with nursing and nurse. Although many of their activities are similar, others are very different; a view highlighted in various reports, shared by the UK Central Council for Nursing, Midwifery and Health Visiting (UKCC 1986a) and acknowledged by Williams (1979).

The pressure to bring the 'professions' together succeeded in 1979 with the passing of the Nurses, Midwives and Health Visitors Act. This was intended to bring all together and to create a better understanding of each other's roles, but it has actually led to a greater degree of alienation. There is a continuing failure to acknowledge nursing and midwifery as separate professions, and resentment that either considers itself different from the other.

These attitudes are reflected by all disciplines at all levels, from the government health departments to practitioners. Unfortunately they have led to a rivalry that is sometimes destructive rather than productive. It may close the mind, so that anything to do with midwifery is rejected by some nurses, and vice versa.

This was borne out by Midgley's study (1988) of the use of nursing models in midwifery, which highlights a range of views, from how models of nursing can be adapted to midwifery to the rejection of anything to do with nursing. In her survey, to which 135 out of 145 midwifery training institutions responded, 70 did not use a nursing model or the nursing process; 24 used a model and the process; 41 used the process only. Of those using a model most used Orem, 'some loosely' and some in combination with others. The success of implementation was not evaluated.

Generally, the widespread use of nursing models in midwifery has been rejected for the following reasons:

- lack of understanding of their value to midwifery;
- perception of nursing as illness- and problem-related, therefore inappropriate to midwifery which is health-related;
- models being an unknown entity: as John Locke, the philosopher, put it, new opinions are always suspected and usually opposed without any other reason than they are not already common;
- models are seen as theoretical ideas imposed from above.

The value of models to midwifery

We may explore this further with a review of two of the most commonly used nursing models and their relevance to midwifery: Roper, Logan and Tierney's model and Orem's model (Roper, Logan & Tierney 1985, Orem 1980).

Orem's model, with its focus on 'self-care' and health, including the care of dependants, is pertinent to midwifery. Individual responsibility is valued, with health education an important aspect of care. Its underlying features are consistent with the role of the midwife, intervening when necessary (particularly during labour) but with a high supportive/educative profile during pregnancy and the postnatal period.

Few mothers would have the eight deficits in the self-care requisites, so an adaptation of these would be necessary. The importance of cultural aspects seems to be excluded, although it may be considered implicit in the partnership approach.

The concepts of Roper, Logan & Tierney's model are relatively simple to understand, unlike the American models and their difficult terminology. The activities of living are a familiar concept: dynamic, constantly changing, affected by psychological and social factors. The model is excellent in relation to physical aspects of care. Social/educational aspects are referred to but do not seem to be as important, although during childbirth these areas, including the cultural aspects, are extremely relevant. A number of adjustments would have to be made to the list of categories and consideration given to the case of the fetus and to pain, which is a normal occurrence during labour. This could help eliminate unnecessary categories and reduce the amount of paperwork.

An understanding of the assumptions on which models are founded is vital, as their selection for practice should be based on the values and beliefs of the practitioners. If existing models are dismissed, practitioners will need to devise their own.

The philosophy implicit in the nursing process is that of individualised care, to which most midwives are committed. However, assessment, planning, implementation and evaluation is an empty approach unless it is based on a model that acts as a framework to guide care. The rejection of models could support the continuation of a task-orientated approach based on the medical model; this could jeopardise continuity of care, affect relationships with the mother and her family and endanger the midwife's autonomy. A process approach to care could overcome some of the deficiencies of the system and prevent the midwife from becoming a 'maternity nurse' incapable of diagnosing, prescribing care or taking responsibility for her actions. Practice needs to be based on midwifery theory, which in turn should be based on a sound evaluation of practice.

A model, therefore, is beneficial to midwifery practice for the following reasons:

- It coordinates the beliefs of midwives about the care they give.
- It enables continuity of care.
- It furthers the giving of consistent advice.
- It improves record-keeping.
- It assists in the identification of poor practice.
- It aids the development of research into midwifery practice.
- It supports the practitioner's autonomy.

A model should help to assist in decision-making about care, building a knowledge base which is open to critical evaluation and thus research. The choice of model depends on many factors, but a consideration of the work of the theorists and some of the principles on which nursing models are founded gives valuable insights. An understanding of the theory is essential to introduce a model but testing it in practice is of paramount importance. Models, although grounded in theory, are basically practical tools and it may be useful to pilot several before choosing one. Different areas require different approaches to care and therefore different models; a neonatal unit concerned with sick babies will make a different choice from a midwifery unit, where the concern is healthy mothers and babies.

Midwives may wish to develop and use a model of nursing as the basis of care. Alternatively, if these models do not fit in with their perceptions and expectations, they may wish to take an eclectic approach, selecting those concepts most suited to midwifery from several models, or they may wish to develop their own. NERU found that failure of implementation followed the imposition of models by managers (Nursing Education Research Unit 1986).

A model for midwifery

The final part of this chapter will concentrate on a model for midwifery, its use in practice, and how it was devised. A number of nursing models were considered, but they failed to address all the issues relevant to midwifery practice in viewing childbirth as a normal physiological process, related to health rather than illness. The midwives wanted to base the model on human needs, and so the work of Maslow (1971) was used. We were assisted in devising a model by the work of Minshull, Ross & Turner (1986), who used Maslow's work as a framework for practice in a nursing setting.

Any model should address four areas: the person receiving care, health, nursing (in this case midwifery), and the context in which care takes place. Figure 7.1 is a diagrammatic representation of the model devised.

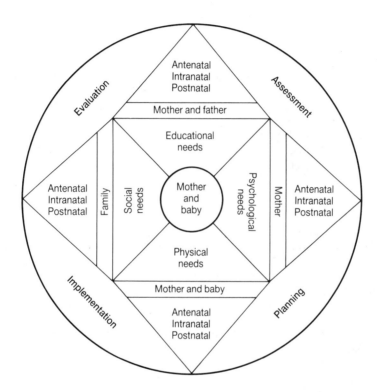

Figure 7.1   A human needs model for midwifery

Mother and baby

The mother and baby are central to the model. All care given by the midwife has the prime purpose of meeting the individual needs of mother and baby. These needs can be categorised into four essential groups: physical; psychological, including spiritual; social; and educational.

Failure to meet the needs of the mother and baby could cause them to regress in all four spheres. In the physical and psychological spheres they may regress from health to illness. In the social sphere they may regress from well-being to disharmony, and in the educational sphere they may regress from a state of confidence to one of insecurity.

Environment

The environment encompasses all situations in which the mother and baby receive care by the midwife, in their antenatal, intranatal and postnatal period. The model can be used effectively by midwives working in an integrated service in hospital and/or community settings.

Health

The model stresses the importance of seeing pregnancy, labour and the puerperium as an altered state of health and not as an illness. The mother and baby, however, have needs that must be met for this healthy state to be maintained. The categories of need are based on Maslow's hierarchy of human needs and emphasise that to maintain health in the mother and baby a sequence of need determination should be followed. A foundation of physical well-being should be laid before psychological, spiritual, social and finally educational well-being can be achieved.

Midwife

The model stresses that the midwife and the mother are partners in care. The midwife, using the process as a tool, will assist the mother in pregnancy, labour and the puerperium to determine her own needs and those of her baby, plan care for herself and the baby, and carry out that care, evaluating the effectiveness in meeting these needs in the four identified areas: physical, psychological, spiritual and social/educational.

   The process enables the model to be put into practice. It also assists in the fulfilment of the European Community directives and complies with the Midwives' Rules (UKCC 1986b, c).

Use of the model in practice

Assessment

A mother-and-baby profile containing information on past history and delivery details will have been completed antenatally. On admission an assessment of the mother and baby, using the four areas identified as the basis of the model, is completed by the midwife. Observations are recorded on the appropriate chart. Thereafter assessment and observations are undertaken as often as necessary.

Planning

Using the assessment as a baseline, problems and/or needs are highlighted and a care plan devised. The problems/needs are prefixed as follows:

A – Physical
B – Psychological, including spiritual
C – Social
D – Educational

This allows the midwife to identify the areas as specified in the model and make them clear on the plan.

Implementation

We can illustrate the assessment and use of the care plan by means of a case study. Mrs Jones, aged 25, gravida 3, experienced no problems during preparation. She attended two preparation for parenthood classes. Epidural analgesia was established early in labour, and labour progressed to a normal delivery of a live boy. The third stage was normal, perineum intact. Mrs Jones bottle-fed her previous offspring but wished to breastfeed this baby.

On admission to the postnatal ward, an assessment was carried out and the records completed as follows:

● *Physical* – Partial sensation in legs and inability to pass urine due to the effects of the epidural analgesia. Otherwise the uterus was well contracted with normal lochial discharges. Baby was put to the breast in delivery suite; colour, tone, behaviour and observations were normal.

● *Psychological* – Interaction with baby at delivery was good.

● *Social* – Father present at delivery; children aged 3 and 5 were being looked after by Mrs Jones' mother.

● *Educational* – She wishes to breastfeed this baby; previous babies were bottle-fed, so she feels a little apprehensive. Parentcraft classes were attended during pregnancy, and the midwife responsible is to be informed of the delivery.

As shown in the care plan (Figure 7.2), only specific needs or problems are identified; all other needs deemed normal are excluded. This makes the planning of care meaningful and less repetitive. A standard care plan may be developed for the purposes of training and for the record in case of litigation. Midwifery practice would be updated taking account of research and the views of those using the maternity services.

Evaluation

A written record is made at the end of each shift, when problems/needs identified on the care plan are reviewed. Evaluation of care as planned is recorded. A column is included for additional information for things that are important but are not evaluations of care. Figure 7.3 is an example relevant to Mrs Jones. Unit policy requires a midwife to indicate the end of a shift period; even where comment is not necessary, a signature and time are recorded.

Observations of Mrs Jones and her baby were recorded on the appropriate charts. As they were perfectly normal they were not referred to on the care plan

Date/time	Problem/need	Midwifery care	Review date/time
12.4.88 10.00	A1 Restricted mobility due to epidural	Observe for return of complete sensation, i.e. able to go to the toilet unassisted	Discretion of midwife, according to findings
	A2 Failure to pass urine	Assist micturition by escorting to toilet Palpate abdomen to ensure: • complete emptying of bladder • uterus well contracted Observe lochial discharge to determine colour and quantity are normal	Discretion of midwife, according to clinical findings
10.00	D1 Anxious about breastfeeding	Breastfeed frequently, the same midwife to supervise each feed where possible	2–3 hourly
23.00	B1 Restless due to 'after'-pains, unable to sleep	Uterus checked to ensure well contracted, and observe that lochial discharges were normal Midwife prescribed paracetamol and temazepam Hot drink given Expressed breast milk to be given for next feed, to allow mother to sleep for longer	Hourly, then 3 hourly

Figure 7.2   Care plan for Mrs Jones

or evaluation sheet. As everything progressed satisfactorily, the only medical staff involvement was the paediatrician, who examined the baby, confirming that he was normal and ready to go home. The midwife and Mrs Jones decided that the most suitable time for transfer home was on the third day, and the community midwife was contacted.

How the model was devised

Figure 7.4 summarises the stages in the development of the midwifery model. It shows a move towards a more individual approach to care, with discussions of the beliefs and values of mothers and midwives being important considerations. It can be seen that a review of existing nursing models was undertaken, but for the reasons given earlier in the text these were rejected in favour of the practitioners developing a model based on their own practice. Lister (1987) suggests that this inductive approach is suited to human sciences, and agrees with

Date	Time	Evaluation of care	Additional information
12.4.88	11.00	A2 Problem solved	Parentcraft midwife informed of admission
	13.30	A1 Sensation returned	
	21.15	D1 Baby suckling well Mother relaxed Still requires supervision	
13.4.88	07.30	D1 Continuing to breastfeed well	Blood taken for haemoglobin
		B1 Slept well between feeds	Community midwife to make arrangements for home transfer
	13.30		Paediatrician to see baby
			Seen 16.00 hours, discharged
	21.15		
14.4.88	07.30	D1 Continues to breastfeed well	
		B1 Sedative not necessary	
	13.30	Seen and examined by midwife	
		To be transferred home when husband able to arrange transport	Haemoglobin 11 g
		Community midwife notified	
		Notes to be taken home by mother for the midwife	

Figure 7.3 Evaluation of care

others that model development should be an ongoing, thought-provoking concern.

Following the identification of a model based on practice, and agreement on using the 'nursing' process, the midwives highlighted the need to review existing documentation. They considered it inappropriate and redesigned the forms, which reduced the paperwork and abolished duplication of information. It is important to note the timescale: planning began in 1984 and culminated in 1988 with a model of care that was capable of realistic application, meaningful in the practice of midwifery, and most importantly 'owned' by the midwives.

A model guides practice, aids coordination of care, and allows critical evaluation of the care given. It affords midwives the opportunity to discuss their values

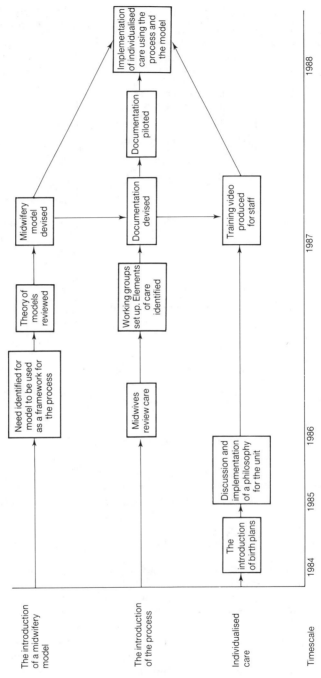

Figure 7.4   Stages in the development of a model for midwifery

and beliefs, thus allowing them to control the care they give. The model presented here reflects the views, philosophies and assumptions of one group of midwives. It is a framework serving as a guide to practice, a structured way to plan, implement and evaluate care. The approach used may appear deficient to the academic, but it was an acceptable way forward for these midwives. It is a basis from which progress can be made, a beginning capable of development. In the words of Winston Churchill:

> 'This is not the end. It is not even the beginning of the end. But it is perhaps the end of the beginning.'

References

Aggleton P & Chalmers H (1986) *Nursing Models and the Nursing Process.* London: Macmillan.

Clifford C (1988) *An Experience of Transition from a Medical Model to a Nursing Model in Nurse Education.* Paper presented at a conference on nursing education, University of Wales.

Davies C (1980) A constant casualty: nurse education in Britain and the USA to 1939. In Davies C, ed., *Rewriting Nursing History*. Beckenham: Croom Helm.

General Nursing Council for England and Wales (1977) *A Statement of Educational Policy.* Circular 77/19/A. London: GNC.

Lister P (1987) The misunderstood model. *Nursing Times,* **83**(41), 40–42.

Maslow A (1971) *Motivation and Personality.* 2nd edn. New York: Harper and Row.

Midgley C (1988) *The Use of Models for Nursing within Midwifery Training Hospitals in England.* Unpublished paper, Huddersfield Polytechnic.

Minshull J, Ross K & Turner J (1986) The human needs model of nursing. *Journal of Advanced Nursing,* **11**(6), 643–649.

Nursing Education Research Unit (1986) *Report of the Nursing Process Evaluation Working Group.* NERU 5. London: King's College.

Orem D (1980) *Nursing: Concepts of Practice.* New York: McGraw-Hill.

Roper N, Logan W & Tierney A (1985) *The Elements of Nursing.* Edinburgh: Churchill Livingstone.

UKCC (1986a) *Project 2000: A New Preparation for Practice.* London: UKCC.

UKCC (1986b) *A Midwife's Code of Practice.* London: UKCC.

UKCC (1986c) *Midwives' Rules.* London: UKCC.

Versluysen M (1980) Old wives' tales? Woman healers in English history. In Davies C, ed., *Rewriting Nursing History.* Beckenham: Croom Helm.

Williams S (1979) Student nurses' attitudes towards midwifery. *Nursing Times,* **75**(14), 41–44.

Models for Nursing 2
Edited by B Kershaw and J Salvage
© 1990 Scutari Press

8

The Value of Models in District Nursing

ANNE JONES

'The profession of nursing is surrounded by myths and beliefs which defy objective examination, because the commonly held belief is that it is impossible to define what nursing actually is. Opinions such as: "British nursing is the best in the world; nursing standards have deteriorated...; nursing is an art based on common sense; nurses know intuitively when what they do is 'good' but it eludes description; nurses are born not made; good nursing students are poor nurse practitioners (and vice versa); nursing can only be learned at the bedside" make it difficult to examine the role of nursing scientifically because, true or false, they are opinions which are accepted uncritically for the most part by a professional group of people.' – SCHRÖCK, 1981.

Recent developments in health care organisation and delivery have made it important for nurses to be able to account for their practice in a precise way. Demand has become more large-scale and complex, and public awareness of health as a right will further increase demand. Although there is no limit to potential demands, the same cannot be said for resources. The community is one of the fastest growing areas of demand due to policies such as earlier discharge from hospital, the closure of mental hospitals, and the maintenance at home of elderly and disabled people who in times past would have remained in institutions. These developments will give rise to changes in the organisation of health care services, to achieve economies of scale while ensuring a fair distribution of resources according to needs (Smith 1981).

The scale and complexity of care in the community is an enormous challenge to health professionals. The setting up of neighbourhoods as recommended in the Cumberlege report (DHSS 1986) will simplify the coordination and delivery of services in a given area. The establishment of efficient primary health care teams, pooling specialist knowledge and skills, would be a less arduous task if the roles of the various disciplines were clearly stated and understood. Clarity of documentation facilitates the recognition by management of growing areas of demand, or inadequacies in existing services, and leads to improvements in future planning and division of resources. Statistically proven demands for growth in community services are more powerful political tools than unsubstantiated observations made by those delivering care.

The population as a whole is ageing. This demographic change is becoming more marked as people live longer while there has been an accompanying drop in the birthrate. Epidemiological changes have also occurred: some diseases that once ravaged whole communities have been conquered, but others have developed to take their place and to demand a larger proportion of nurses' attention. Chronic illness has replaced acute illness as a priority health problem, including circulatory diseases, cancer, and diseases and disabilities of old age as well as those affected by individual behaviour. Technical skills in saving lives and dealing with medical emergencies are of little use in the care of patients who will not recover, but who need considerable nursing care to enable them to live full and useful lives.

Caring for the chronically sick demands health teaching and psychological skills which are relatively new to nursing. The district nurse must learn her patients' family dynamics and motivation, and develop techniques and strategies to help them live with their illness. Some chronic illnesses may be difficult to manage and may require much health teaching and counselling in addition to more traditional skills. The elderly have special needs; although illness and disability are not essential concomitants of old age, their incidence is higher than among the general population and the level of dependence is greater. Health professionals must avoid the stereotyping and stigma attached to old age, and ensure that the care of the elderly is not goalless, and that quality of life is assured.

The care of terminally ill people at home is a growing and demanding part of the district nurse's workload. It involves the development of new skills to understand pain control, dietary requirements and psychological needs of the dying patient, family and carers. The complex delivery of care involves the contributions of the general practitioner, nurse, social worker, chaplain, occupational therapist and physiotherapist, and requires much discussion, assessment and interchange of ideas. Clarity of the individual role is essential for good team management (Copp 1981).

The nurse is often in a position of running to keep up with the challenges of needing to know what is going on and needing to care for patients in wholly changed circumstances. Needs can remain unmet in the rush to complete other tasks. Nurses' practice is determined not only by patients' needs and medical diagnostic or therapeutic demands, but by the setting in which the care is delivered. Patients are not automatically compliant, and must be helped to understand why following a course of treatment is necessary. They may not accept a half-thought-through explanation in patient teaching when they have watched a television programme on their condition and know more about it than their nurse.

Illness-orientated medical care is no longer always sufficient, and is perhaps not appropriate for many of our patients' problems. Ways must be found to make better use of scarce health manpower, to improve access to and quality of care and simultaneously to decrease costs.

Nursing models and the multidisciplinary approach

To meet all the challenges and changes of nursing in modern times, the profession must be open to examination and research. Traditionally there has been no documentation to allow the scrutiny of nursing principles and theory; neglect of theory and obsession with 'doing' have meant that there is no commonly accepted model. The need to yoke together separate but interlinked professional skills has arisen over the last 20 years in response to the growth in the complexity of services, the expansion of knowledge and the subsequent increase in specialisation. One person may suffer from limitations of knowledge or experience, but a team of different but interrelated workers can wipe out these deficiencies (Hunt 1983).

Most people receive health care from more than one type of worker. A team is more than a collection of individuals; it implies that a number of people are working cooperatively to achieve a common goal. The composition of the team will depend on the individual needs of the client or patient, but the recipient of care must remain its most important component. Each member has a special contribution to make, though certain actions may overlap. All operate from different but complementary models for practice; all members of practice disciplines have some sort of 'model' in their heads and though there may be personal variations, occupational groups usually share a common understanding of their own discipline. Explicit models for practice iron out personal differences and allow individuals to participate effectively in the multidisciplinary team. The all too common problem of nurses' inability to become equal members of the team may partly be overcome by the nurses agreeing on an appropriate practice model and then making this explicit to the other disciplines. Their contribution will not be valued and their expertise will be underused if they are not able to establish their particular role in the team (Pearson 1986).

The variety in client groups and the settings in which they require care makes the universal use of an all-embracing nursing model impossible. An abundance of models specific to nursing is now available from which one can be chosen to suit almost any field. Each team of nurses, whether on a ward or in the community, should find it possible to agree on a model that reflects for them the reality of their practice.

The model can be used to describe the way in which nurses practise in clear, straightforward and confident terms. Such a statement will increase understanding of the nurse's role among the team members and will lead them to value nursing more. The improved use of nursing skills will benefit nurses, and efficient working of the team will ensure quality for the patient.

Most studies of interdisciplinary teamwork have concluded that the majority of teams are working at levels well below what is possible. Those involved must work together and coordinate their activities, since the job cannot be done by one person alone. This is not to say that each task must be tackled by all members simultaneously, but that at various times the nature of the task will require coordinating, to schedule work, allocate priorities and share information as a basis for problem-sharing and decision-making. Problems related to teamwork do not appear to be inherent in all methods of working, but seem to be associated with the extent to which team members' roles and functions are clearly defined and complement each other. Role ambiguity and conflict compound the problems (Hunt 1983).

Putting models into practice

The use of a nursing model in the community has enormous potential as a teaching tool, not only helping student district nurses to learn about nursing in the community, but also assisting students on the basic training programme when they accompany district nurses as observers. Methods of assessing patients in their home environment can be demonstrated. Should the format already be familiar to them from the hospital setting, they will readily identify with it, providing an exercise in the transfer of learning. Other students who require an insight into district nursing, such as health visitors, social work students or GP trainees, could be helped to learn in a similar manner (Roper, Logan & Tierney 1983).

It is not sufficient simply to encourage a nurse or group of nurses to use a model for practice. The plethora of models now available presents a bewildering choice to those unfamiliar with their use. In some areas the nursing process has not long been introduced and nurses are understandably reluctant to embrace what they perceive as yet another new method in the delivery of care. Before they can choose a model to practise from, nurses need opportunities to explore the options and to discuss their own ideas. Understanding models and the reasons for their use is easier in groups, where there is pooling of ideas and interpretation; meetings for staff to study various approaches can be productive. Updating courses for all qualified nurses are necessary to familiarise them with models, and guidance should then be given on the choice of a suitable model. Special attention should be given to practical work teachers to enable them to give the necessary support to students. Suitable documentation is essential to facilitate the use of a particular model, and support and encouragement from management is desirable at all stages in its introduction.

Apart from encouraging improved standards of patient care, an analysis of the records used in a nursing model will add to that body of knowledge which is *nursing* – essential for any research-based profession, as indicated in the Briggs report (Committee on Nursing 1972).

Case study using Orem's self-care model

Michael Mitchell was referred to me by his GP who explained that he was suffering from cancer of the head of the pancreas with liver secondaries. He had recently been discharged from hospital and did not know his condition was terminal. The GP had not had confirmation from the hospital of the terminal nature of the illness, but was surmising it from the summary of the surgery he underwent.

I visited Michael at home on 22 February. He answered the door and my first impressions were of an anxious, emaciated man. He seemed surprised at my presence, was not very communicative, and insisted that he did not require nursing services of any kind. It was difficult to elicit personal details such as any symptoms he was experiencing or the quality of his diet, but he insisted he was symptom-free and was 'getting better'. I decided to visit him weekly in the hope of building up a relationship that would enable nursing services to be given.

Michael was 46 and unmarried. He had come from Ireland the previous summer to stay with his sister and attend a niece's wedding. He had been taken ill shortly afterwards, and apart from his hospital admissions had lived with his sister and her husband ever since. He expected to be well enough to return to Ireland within a couple of months. There was no telephone in the house and he did not know his sister's work number. I supplied him with phone numbers where I could be contacted.

Four days later I had a call from Michael's sister, who wanted to come to see me. She did not want Michael to be present, so I suggested we should meet at the clinic where I am based. This interview proved very productive. Two women arrived – both his sisters. They were very worried about him, and had only recently been informed by the GP of the expected outcome. They said that since all the family were in full employment it would not be possible to care for Michael at home when his condition deteriorated. I explained about the district nursing and Macmillan services, and the local hospice. They expressed a preference for a Catholic hospice they knew, though since this was further away and less convenient they were undecided about it.

The sisters explained that Michael had no income, since he was unemployed and the benefits he drew in Ireland were only payable while he was resident there. Significantly, they told me how Michael cared for their father who had died 'of the same thing' several years before and whose final months had not been comfortable. They felt that Michael would be unable to cope with the information that his condition was terminal, though following discussion they agreed that it was desirable that he should be told, should the opportunity arise. Since they said that his appetite was very poor I gave them samples of fortified foods and told them how to apply for a prescription exemption.

The picture emerging was that although Michael professed to be capable of caring for himself, his relatives saw him as being in need of assistance. His prognosis made it clear that his self-care needs would rapidly outstrip his ability to meet them. Already his diet was inadequate; he remained at home alone most of the day, in bed or sitting in a chair, and his emaciation made pressure sores a real possibility. His sisters were anxious and nervous about the possibility of providing care, saying that he needed 'professional' care. I felt sure this was why admission to a hospice seemed a good solution to them. The memories of their father's final illness made them worried that Michael was destined to suffer intractable pain.

To begin to devise a care plan for Michael, it was necessary to build up a relationship with him and to help him to maintain his independence as much as possible. I visited him weekly for the next month and gradually he began to admit to pain and nausea. After discussion with the GP he started taking 30 mg sustained release morphine twice a day and 10 mg metoclopramide three times a day. It took a week to convince him to take the morphine every 12 hours whether pain was present or not; after that the pain was controlled but nausea remained troublesome. His appetite was poor and he did not like my food samples. Opportunities were sought to discuss his condition, but he remained uncommunicative and determinedly optimistic. After four weeks he felt too ill to attend an outpatient appointment, and requested hospital admission.

Progress had been very slow during this period. Michael was withdrawn and reluctant to admit to any symptoms. There was no opportunity to get to know other family members as they were out at work. Michael's failure to accept his illness appeared the greatest barrier to the implementation of a plan that would enable him to meet at least some of his self-care requisites. I hoped that while he was in hospital he would be informed of his diagnosis and prognosis.

He stayed in hospital for three weeks and was discharged in a much weaker state. His emaciation was extreme and he had become even more uncommunicative. No-one had spoken to him about his condition or future. He was more or less bed-bound. His medications had been changed. Nausea and vomiting were a persistent problem and his appetite was very poor, though he tolerated a home-made liquid food recommended by the hospital dietician. He was still resistant to nursing care, but allowed me to apply an occlusive dressing to a small sacral sore and to order a sheepskin for his bed. His wishes to be self-caring were respected as far as possible, but I started daily visits.

Michael's sister could see that his condition was deteriorating, and she became anxious about the future. Hospice admission was discussed and the family thought this was the best option until I explained that Michael would need to know his diagnosis, as this was a requirement for hospice admission. The problem was discussed with the GP who agreed with the proposed plan and visited Michael on several occasions hoping to find an opportunity to discuss the future with him. However, he found him as withdrawn as I did and no progress was made.

By this time it had become apparent that Michael's family was a large one – he had five sisters, two brothers and several cousins, all living within a 40-mile radius, and all aware of what was happening to him. Opinion was divided on whether he should know the outcome of his illness, but it was the subject of much family discussion. They found him irritable and felt uncomfortable in his presence, but were deeply concerned for him and anxious for him to be admitted to the hospice.

The issue of whether to tell or not to tell a patient that his illness is terminal is extremely complex, and there are no hard and fast rules for all patients. Each person has his own method of coping with such knowledge, and it takes time and sensitivity to get to know a patient well enough to decide what they require. In Michael's case, given his severe withdrawal and the very short time left to him, it clearly might not be possible to wait for him to make the first approach. He avoided asking questions of the nurses or doctor but expressed his fears to his family, who felt unable to deal with them. I thought referral to the Macmillan nurses would be beneficial, since their visits could be much longer than those of the district nurse.

Michael's worsening nausea and vomiting refused to respond to thrice daily prochlorperazine 10mg and domperidone suppositories. This finally gave me the opportunity to introduce the Macmillan nurse. I explained to him that she might be able to suggest medication to control his nausea, and he agreed to see her. This was a significant stage in his progress, as following her first visit he finally knew what his condition was. He asked her, 'How long do I have?' and said he had realised what his condition was when he was not given any treatment in hospital. The anxieties of his family were quickly allayed when they saw the change in his expression and mood. More discussion followed and it was decided that he should remain at home; relatives would take turns to care for him daily.

The fact that Michael was now fully informed about his condition removed one of the greatest difficulties for the relatives. They were not only willing but eager to look after him, and after this the hospice was no longer mentioned. With help and advice they now provided some care, and Michael accepted nursing care less reluctantly. A Spenco mattress, commode and urinal were ordered and oral swabs supplied. He gradually allowed the nurses to take over his care. Medication was monitored daily and changed after discussion with the GP and Macmillan nurse. The family dispensed it as Michael found the frequent changes confusing. He did not want to see the social worker about his finances and the family did not feel it appropriate to request the chaplain to visit. He remained uncommunicative with the nurses, but feedback from the family suggested that he was happy with his care. New suggestions were discussed with him, and the family, and usually accepted. He did not often speak openly of what was happening, but he seemed more relaxed and the family felt comfortable with him again. He did not want to see a priest at this stage, though he did talk about his house and what would happen to it after his death.

Towards the end of April his condition worsened. Pain and nausea were difficult to control but were monitored constantly. The use of a syringe driver was discussed. The evening nursing service was asked to start visiting, and Michael requested to see a priest. Over the next few days he grew very weak. The use of a syringe driver was started and nursing visits increased. A night sitter from the Marie Curie service was offered, but family members remained with him constantly and felt this was unnecessary. In mid-May following a day of Cheyne – Stokes respirations, Michael died in the presence of his family two days after his 47th birthday.

A month later the Macmillan nurse and I visited Michael's family. They told us about his funeral in Ireland, discussed their feelings about their brother's last months, and expressed satisfaction with the outcome. They admitted to reservations about whether Michael should have known his diagnosis, but in retrospect they felt this knowledge had enabled him to meet death with dignity, and said their own views on death and dying had changed a great deal as a result. They all felt that he had better care than they realised was available, and were glad that he had not been taken ill in Ireland where he would have been alone and they would not have been able to care for him.

Postscript

In many health authorities like my own, nursing models for practice are not yet used in the community except by personally motivated nurses. Ideas of what constitutes good nursing care are as diverse as the people who give the service.

The nursing process is used with varying degrees of efficiency. Pooling of ideas and opinions would help to standardise the quality of nursing care and to clarify the future development of district nursing services at a time when demands are growing at an alarming pace. The use of nursing models is one way of community nursing. Nevertheless it requires considerable time, dedication, commitment and support, both moral and financial, to introduce such a radical change in practice when existing services are stretched to the limit.

References

Committee on Nursing (1972) *Report of the Committee on Nursing* (the Briggs report). London: HMSO.

Copp L (1981) Significant issues in nursing gerontology. In Hockey L, ed., *Current Issues in Nursing*. Edinburgh: Churchill Livingstone.

Department of Health and Social Security (1986) *Neighbourhood Nursing – a Focus for Care. Report of the Community Nursing Review in England.* London: HMSO.

Hunt M (1983) Possibilities and problems of interdisciplinary teamwork. In Clark J & Henderson J, eds, *Community Health.* Edinburgh: Churchill Livingstone.

Pearson A (1986) Nursing models and multidisciplinary teamwork. In Kershaw B & Salvage J, eds, *Models for Nursing.* Chichester: John Wiley.

Roper N, Logan & Tierney A (1983) *Using a Model for Nursing.* Edinburgh: Churchill Livingstone.

Schröck R (1981) Philosophical issues. In Hockey L, ed., *Current Issues in Nursing.* Edinburgh: Churchill Livingstone.

Smith J (1981) Issues in nursing administration. In Hockey L, ed., *Current Issues in Nursing.* Edinburgh: Churchill Livingstone.

Models for Nursing 2
Edited by B Kershaw and J Salvage
© 1990 Scutari Press

9

Mental Handicap and Nursing Models

CHRIS ELLIOTT-CANNON

Mental handicap nursing has made enormous strides in the last decade. A new syllabus, new settings for practice and new ways of working have transformed a committed but largely institutionalised staff group into a dynamic professional enterprise at the forefront of many developments.

Insights from many fields have been incorporated into the ethos and practice of mental handicap nursing. From the human rights movement has come a philosophy, 'normalisation', which, despite the difficulties of the term, has led to a new, comprehensive set of values on which to base practice. From psychology has come a scientific approach to behaviour and the adoption of behavioural skills as an important tool in the mental handicap nurse's repertoire. Social work has given us a new understanding of the importance of the family as a focal influence on the individual and vice versa; also of casework skills. From psychiatry, notions of therapy, including family therapy and therapeutic use of self, have helped to shape a new style of work. The field of education has given nurses curriculum-building theory and teaching skills, to be applied to individuals and to groups.

The concept of care, holism and a constructive blend of genericism with specialism is perhaps better demonstrated in this field than in any other. The synthesis of these theoretical and practical approaches with the experience and commitment of mental handicap nurses is already substantial, and the process of translating this new synthesis into practice and service contexts is well advanced.

Much remains to be done, however, in two particular areas: developing service patterns that facilitate the use of all that has been achieved, and incorporating the valuable new perspectives now emanating from mainstream nursing much more fully into mental handicap nursing. Applying theory and models is a good example.

Developing new service patterns

The move to community care has been led by the field of mental handicap. The change from largely medical models of care to largely social models has had an unfortunate consequence: although nurses are keen to work in any setting and in non-medical ways, they are still perceived by others as 'hospital' staff. In many places nurses are valued and active in community settings, often leading developments, but in others they are excluded. A dogmatic pursuit of one inter-pretation of community care is developing (often for partisan reasons); com-munity care is being equated with 'local authority' care, and local authority care is equated with social workers, not nurses.

Since the Jay report (DHSS 1979) the word 'normalisation' has been assumed to mean normal services, which in turn is interpreted by many as generic social services. Certainly Jay stressed the need for every person with a mental handicap to have access to all services and rights enjoyed by fellow citizens and to have non-labelling service provision. It also said, however, that many people with a mental handicap need special services, but there are signs that such services are being hindered in their development by empire-building and professional rivalry, to the detriment of people with mental handicaps. Progress is also hampered by the failure of important reports (Audit Commission 1986, DHSS 1988) to recognise the need for health authorities and mental handicap nurses to participate fully in service developments. Mental handicap community care is a multidisciplinary business, not a unidisciplinary one.

Some of the new plans and developments sadly refuse to accept a health authority or nursing presence. If nurses are employed, they are at best 'seconded' to the local authority, and often they are not employed as nurses. Social service departments, reluctantly accepting that nurses have useful skills, are nevertheless expecting them to shed their nursing identity, which is damaging to their profes-sional self-esteem and to the maintenance of the skills, knowledge and contacts that made them valuable in the first place. The dilution of the nursing connection would remove them from the current developments in nursing theory, practice, education and updating; and would lose supervision and management by nurses, that is by those best qualified to facilitate and reinforce the use of nursing skills and perspectives.

There are many external reasons for this state of affairs, compounded by an important internal factor. Mental handicap nurses during the 1970s were caught in the trap of confusing social models of care with social service patterns of service. Their lack of conviction that 'nursing' was an appropriate description for them or their activities, at the very time when discharge plans and new service developments were being discussed, led to compliance with an emphasis on transfer to local authority and 'social work' care.

The notion that nursing is really about caring for sick people has been the root of the problem. Once the new emphasis on holistic care and promotion of health and independence gained a grip, the atmosphere changed. While normalisation was helping to provide a values base, however, there was still no clear conceptual framework for mental handicap nursing care. Such frameworks are available in nursing models: the full exploration and development of models as conceptual structures for this speciality is a fascinating issue.

Models and mental handicap nursing

Most mental handicap nurses have only recently heard about models of nursing, which are still largely seen as something general nursing colleagues do. Where they are used, it is usually by students trying out new approaches to structuring care, with varying degrees of guidance and understanding on the part of all concerned. Most of the models are American and have arisen from the thinking of nurses working with general or psychiatric patients; the case examples are drawn from those fields. Although there is a wealth of literature about models and their use, there are few examples of detailed application in mental handicap.

The notion of a model in a general sense is familiar in mental handicap, where years of fighting the 'institutional model', the 'medical model' and the 'custodial model' have led to an emphasis on 'social models', 'behavioural models' and 'ordinary life models'. These are all snapshot terms, which each cover a set of concepts in relation to each other. For example, an ordinary life model includes a number of concepts. Human beings are to be 'valued'; one's 'home' should be in 'ordinary surroundings'. Notions of 'independence', 'community,' 'habilitation' and 'rehabilitation' are implicit. Each concept gives us ideas about both the goals to be chosen and ways of working.

Similarly, a model of nursing is simply a set of related concepts, applicable to nursing, which provide a mental snapshot or 'hook' on which to focus one's approach and work. We all have a personal model which involves ideas, beliefs, knowledge and experience. This may be clear or vague and influences our practice either consciously or subconsciously. We need to explore our own model and other models in order to see how they relate to each other and to make explicit what is sometimes implicit (Pearson & Vaughan 1986). It is particularly important that we share this analysis with colleagues.

How does the nursing process differ from nursing models? The nursing process approach is well known in mental handicap, although, sadly, not always well used. It is a central part of our thinking, yet its relationship to models is often confused, although the difference is really very clear. Nursing process is the systematic device that enables nurses to put into practice any nursing model. The nursing process on its own is not enough. It is a scientific process or method, a systematic way of approaching a job. It uses management terminology to tackle needs and problems but it has no philosophical basis, no inherent goals, no view of human nature, no clue about the nature of nursing. Models, by contrast, provide a rationale for caring interventions (Barber 1987). They are not just academic playthings; although academics have helped to clarify theory and concepts to the advantage of practitioners, it is practitioners who use them and for whom models are a tool to guide actions.

What are the special features and concepts of a nursing model? Models for any discipline will draw on theory and concepts. In nursing, these include systems theory, development theory, and interactionist theory. Theories can interrelate concepts in such a way as to create a different perspective of a particular phenomenon (George 1985). Theories are constructed from concepts, which are abstract ideas or mental images representing reality. Concepts basic and common to all nursing theories include person, environment, health and nursing (Young 1987). Every model should say something about these four concepts, which provide its building blocks; here they will be examined in relation to mental handicap.

Person

The concept of the person refers to all human beings. Nurses have traditionally emphasised the biological properties of people and their diseases and disabilities. As the social sciences developed, mind–body relationships were increasingly stressed and nurses became more concerned with the psychological aspects of behaviour, particularly human status as a bio-psychosocial being. The belief in the integrated nature of the person and hence the need to approach care in a way which recognises that perception is summed up in the idea of 'holism'.

Recently there has been a growing understanding of the centrality of the interactions of the person with other people, family, community and environment. The notion of humanism is also important. Most nursing models emphasise a belief in the nature of people as intrinsically motivated or capable of being motivated, intrinsically valued and entitled to quality of life and respect. In mental handicap these three notions of holism, interaction and humanism are well understood.

The idea of holism perhaps provides one of the main reasons for the mental handicap nurse's existence. By claiming to care for the person as a whole person, using knowledge and skills relevant to biological, psychological and social needs, the nurse is offering something unique to the client – holistic insight and care. There is also a clear trend towards recognition that people with a mental handicap have their own self-concept, emotional life and emotional and interaction needs. Finally, the nursing concept of the person contains an inherent belief that everyone has rights and worth as a human being capable of development. This belief, incorporated in the notion of humanism, implies that each client has the right to skilled nursing, advocacy, choice and dignity, and a scientific, caring approach to him as a valued person.

Environment

'The person is in a constant state of action and reaction with the environment' (Wright 1986). The environment includes internal and external physical, emotional and social factors, but this has not always been recognised. Early in the history of the National Health Service the emphasis was on public health and the physical environment, and the external environment was stressed in early mental handicap care. Early definitions of normalisation, for example, talked of 'normalisation of the conditions' or 'providing normalised environments' (Grunewald 1972). The emphasis lay on the physical environment of furniture and equipment: Gunzburg's inventory for assessing the quality of care, the '39 steps', consisted mostly of a list of fittings (1970).

Later, with the growth in understanding of physiological and pathological processes of disease and health, the concept was expanded to include a person's internal environment: not only did the external physical environment influence people and their behaviour, but so did internal bodily and psychological processes. The environment is now both internal and external, physical, psychological and social. In mental handicap the development of the concept of normalisation paralleled this trend. From the early work of Barton (1950) on effects of institutions to the dehumanisation categories of PASS (Program Analysis of Service Systems), there is a clear and growing awareness of the many subtle influences of environment, including a recognition of the intangible influences of interpersonal behaviour and social factors in terms of the total environment and its consequence. One nursing definition is that of Neuman (1974), who described the internal and external environment as intrapersonal, interpersonal and extrapersonal – terms familiar to those who have studied educational psychology.

Health

Health is sometimes conceived of as a continuum ranging from peak wellness to death. Others see it in terms of behavioural stability (King 1971); adaptation (Roy 1984); wholeness (Orem 1971); system stability (Neuman 1974); expressions of life processes (Rogers 1970); and behavioural equilibrium and independent functioning (Johnson 1980). In mental handicap, clients have traditionally been perceived as sick, dangerous, burdens on society, or everlasting children (Wolfensberger 1972). None of these perceptions conveys an image of 'health', yet in physical and mental terms most mentally handicapped people are as healthy as their non-handicapped peers. Disability, handicap and disease should not be confused, as the way we see these notions influences our approach and our attitudes. Mental handicap is not a disease, it is a disability usually only apparent as a 'learning difficulty'. 'Handicap' is a social construct, and people are only as handicapped as their society defines them. A person can have a disability yet be perfectly healthy and in a state of homeostasis.

Health is an individual perception formed from cultural expectations and personal value systems, so it needs to be defined in relation to both humankind and the client. The World Health Organisation declares that health is a complete state of physical, psychological and social well-being (1961), but it may be difficult to find people who consistently match this ideal. All facets of health must be related to society and the individual. A person paralysed in a road accident may work, marry and live a full life. Is he unhealthy? A person with controlled epilepsy may be a member of parliament. A person with a mental handicap may happily live in a supported community group home, and may be enjoying a lifestyle seen by her acquaintances as healthy and worthwhile. Health as a focus of nursing in mental handicap involves not just prevention of potential problems like ill health, or the alleviation of existing ones like the constraints of slow learning. It involves the positive promotion of strategies for achieving physical, personal and social integration as an individual, within a group and in the community at large.

Nursing

As with the other concepts, 'nursing' consists of several important sub-concepts. In mental handicap these include 'care', 'rehabilitation', 'therapy', 'development' and 'independence'. The definition of mental handicap nursing in the national training syllabus includes some of these concepts: 'The function of the nurse for people with mental handicap is directly and skilfully to assist the individual and his family, whatever the handicap, in the acquisition, development and maintenance of those skills that given the necessary ability could be performed unaided; and to do this in such a way as to enable independence to be gained as rapidly and fully as possible, in an environment that maintains a quality of life that would be acceptable to fellow citizens of the same age'. Few of these implicit concepts or tasks are unique to mental handicap nursing, but 'nursing becomes unique by the unique way it combines these features' (Wright 1986). This combination of knowledge, historical experience and current practice results in a body of knowledge which is distinctively nursing.

A definition of nursing should prescribe the role of nurses as they interact with their clients. Terms like 'client', despite their inadequacies, reflect a belief in the recipient of care as a valued person receiving a service in which they have at least equal rights, and a valued role and status. This approach is strong in mental handicap nursing. Ways of working and terminology should avoid labelling in a way that suggests deviancy or inferior status, and should attempt to increase personal competence, integration and community status.

The five 'accomplishments' suggested by O'Brien (1981) provide a useful approach to the role of mental handicap nurses. No model of nursing in mental handicap would be complete without strong evidence of due regard for these aspects of human life.

The five accomplishments

- *Protection of individual rights (choice)* – a service is effective if people are treated with respect and helped to increase their own interests and autonomy.

- *Community presence* – a service is effective if it attends to the location of a service, how people are grouped and the ways in which activities are conducted.

- *Community participation* – is it designed and delivered to increase opportunities to be active with other members of the community in all kinds of community settings?

- *Competence-building* – does it use well-disciplined and systematic methods to improve personal skills in meaningful ways?

- *Community status (respect)* – a service is effective if it actively promotes a positive reputation for users of the service.

Carle has suggested a further accomplishment (1984):

● *Personal continuity* – a service is effective if services are coordinated to support, not supplant, natural relationships in natural settings.

These accomplishments combined with the syllabus definition include two powerful notions. The first is that the individual should be valued, and that developing competency and integration is a key. The second is that nursing skills can and should be directed to those ends.

The chosen role of nursing will be influenced by the definition of the four concepts basic to all nursing models. These concepts are closely interrelated and each model explains the relationship differently. The nurse will be involved on several fronts at the same time. For example, while teaching a client to feed himself, she will be aware of the *social* influences such as the groupings of clients at tables; the external *environmental* influences such as the temperature, noise level and arrangement of furniture; internal environmental factors such as the physical health of the individual and his mood; and *interpersonal* factors such as how she and he feel about each other.

These environmental factors will, in turn, be affected by the nurse's view of *nursing*: how she sees her role and status, and what knowledge, insight and skill she possesses. Her perception of the nature of handicap and health will also influence her role performance and the targets and priorities she sets. Finally, her view of the *person* is vital and will make the difference between a caring but custodial approach, a relatively uncaring and functional approach, and an optimistic view of the client in tune with humanistic notions of intrinsic worth and possibilities. The latter is more likely to lead to a developmental approach to the job, which is a feature of a number of models.

Which model should the mental handicap nurse choose?

A brief introduction such as this can barely begin to explore the growing range of models in relation to mental handicap. No thinking professional can ignore any approach that might improve nursing and client care. Mental handicap nurses can benefit by thinking about and using models of nursing which, with or without adaptation, may improve their practice. Models exist 'to organise nursing as a coherent whole' (Wright 1986). This then is the first major benefit – organisation of care. The nursing process and the individual programme plan are themselves only planning or action devices – worthwhile in themselves, but containing little or no philosophy, little guidance as to why things are done and little to draw the strands together in a logical way.

A second major value of nursing models is that they help to clarify areas of concern such as the nature of people and of their handicaps; the analysis and use of environmental influences; and the relationship between nursing and the role of the mental handicap nurse. All are the subject of a growing body of literature and discussion, but tend to be seen in isolation from each other. Models of nursing facilitate exploration of the interrelationships, and they must be seen not as rigid formulae but as ways of thinking. They can prompt us to think in new ways about old problems. Finally, as Benner notes (1984), models can act as a map for practice. This excludes the idea that models are alien entities grafted on to existing practice, and assumes that the 'landmarks' (the raw material of ideas, values, experiences) already exist – the map merely articulates them and makes them plain.

Roper, Logan and Tierney's model

Roper, Logan and Tierney's model (1980) appears to be based largely on Henderson's (1966) concept of nursing as assisting and supporting individuals. Her description of activities of living in which nurses can assist, and her emphasis on encouraging independence are familiar to the mental handicap nurse. Roper, Logan and Tierney's model, probably the best known in mental handicap, is the first British attempt at a conceptual model for nursing, and can provide a useful starting point. It sees human beings essentially as seeking self-fulfilment and independence, and mind and body as inseparable. Health is not defined but is seen as independent functioning in 12 pivotal activities of living (ALs) which all people engage in as part of life, living and growing. It is linked to levels of dependence in relation to circumstances.

Each activity of living has many dimensions, e.g. 'life span' (from conception to death) and 'dependency' (total dependence to total independence).

The 12 ALs are a focus, not a separate entity. Each has internal relationships and also interrelates with the other ALs, and each has three components – physiological, social and psychological. The effects of environment and circumstances are recognised as also affecting the capacity to become independent in the ALs. For example, poor living conditions or lack of sensory stimulation can play a part in the development of 'personal cleansing' or 'communicating'. Severe intellectual handicap may adversely affect the ability to 'work and play', and severe physical handicap may affect the potential to control body functions like 'elimination' or 'mobility'.

Nursing activities are regarded as having varied priorities, but Maslow's hierarchy of needs (1943) is seen to be a useful guide, with biological needs often but not always taking priority. Nursing is said to have four components: the 12 ALs and three types of activity. The three types of activity are preventing, comforting and seeking. See Table 9.1 for some examples in a mental handicap context.

The distinctions between physiological, psychological and social components cannot be rigid, but are all intertwined. Similarly, there is considerable overlap and interaction between the preventing, comforting and seeking aspects. Activities like personal cleansing can involve comforting and seeking elements.

The model has several advantages. Its relevance to clients is easily defined, as often some are highly dependent in some ALs and quite able in others. The concepts of 'independence continuums' and the 'life span' approach to long-term care and relationships, the norm in mental handicap, are very useful. Strengths as well as needs can easily be incorporated in the assessment process, and goals and nursing actions can easily be devised.

The disadvantages of the approach are that little is said about the nature of the person, making it easy to use the activities of living approach mechanistically. (This danger could be reduced by an equality of emphasis on psychological

Table 9.1 Mental handicap nursing activities (after Roper, Logan & Tierney 1980)

Activity of living	Client need example	Nursing action (and goal)
Preventing Personal cleansing	Cleanse self	Physiological – encourage handwashing and dressing Psychological – praise warmly Social – encourage peer support (prompt hygiene, relationship and social acceptance)
Maintaining a safe environment	Cross road safely	Physiological – move quickly and safely Psychological – learn rules of road Social – respond to road users (preserve life, develop achievement, promote independence/integration)
Comforting Mobility	Reduce discomfort caused by cerebral palsy	Physiological – give passive movements Psychological – demonstrate caring understanding Social – encourage suitable group activities (alleviate physical/mental discomfort, promote involvement in world)
Seeking Working and playing	Find friends	Physiological – ensure exercise, hygiene, diet Psychological – teach necessary word recognition Social – group learning of social skills (encourage relationships, occupation and self-concept formation)

and social components.) Also, it could become just another checklist with the activities of living seen as too discrete; this would lead to categorising of needs separately rather than seeing them as overlapping and often indivisible. The family and environment are also insufficiently highlighted, and there is too much emphasis on physiological factors.

We need to start by seeing the client as a whole person. If the nurse does this and is aware of the intention of the model, of its advantages and disadvantages, it could be a useful framework for guiding actions.

Johnson's model

In this model (Johnson 1980) the person (a bio-psychosocial being) is seen as having a set of eight interrelated behavioural subsystems, each striving for balance and equilibrium within itself. The person is seen as interacting with the physical and social environment; health is the achievement of a homeostatic but dynamic stability, which includes independent functioning and the notion of adaptation. The subsystems are the affiliative, the aggressive, the eliminative, the ingestive, the restorative and the sexual subsystems. Each continuously motivates the behaviour of the person towards some goal. This set of behavioural subsystems gives mental handicap nurses a clear guide for direct care based on human needs with the intention of promoting a 'stable state'. Nursing involves protection, nurturance and stimulation. Behavioural equilibrium in terms of mental handicap does not mean stasis (stagnation) but optimal functioning, and therefore implies striving towards maximum potential.

Roy's model

This sees the human as a bio-psychosocial 'adaptive' being (Roy 1984). Four modes – physiological, self-concept, role function and interdependence – are the focus of care. Nursing action concentrates on the identification and use of stimuli to support and promote adaptation. This model has much to offer the mental handicap nurse. Although Roy's earlier writings used examples from medical settings, she specifically mentions its use with mentally handicapped children. It is easy to see how concepts like adaptation, role function and interdependence could be applied to handicapped people generally, especially when resettlement is putting more emphasis on changing roles and interdependence, not only for mental handicap nurses but for their clients. The use of stimuli, applied in a caring and scientifically organised way, is also an approach that meshes well with current practice.

Orem's model

Orem sees the human as a bio-psychosocial self-care being who is in interaction with internal and external stimuli (1971). The goal of nursing is supporting the human drive towards optimal functioning. Nursing action centres on three systems: wholly compensatory, partially compensatory and supportive–developmental. Here again, mental handicap nurses can easily understand this set of terms. The essence of mental handicap nursing is to compensate where the disability results in lack of functioning, and to support and develop where there is any possibility of progress towards independence and self-care.

Other models

King's interaction model is another valuable approach (King 1971). Like Peplau (1952) it stresses the paramount importance of relationships, which is highly relevant to mental handicap nursing.

The models most likely to be of value are those which contain concepts like nurturance, stimulation, independence and self-care. These should ring loud bells in mental handicap nurses' minds. Many would respond enthusiastically to the idea of using such models as a framework for their caring and competency work. Suitable opportunities for exploration and discussion of these ideas are essential.

As Roy says, 'a scientific approach to nursing, blended with an increasing understanding of the caring art of nursing, is essential to being able to affect people's health positively in an understandable and consistent way' (Roy 1984). Just as there are the five As (accomplishments) in normalisation, there are five As in nursing models. If you don't like a nursing model, add to it, amend it, abandon it, replace it with your alternative, but don't be apathetic. The use of models in mental handicap is at the beginning, but the field is ripe for development.

References

Audit Commission for Local Authorities in England and Wales (1986) *Making a Reality of Community Care.* London: HMSO.

Barber P, ed. (1987) *Mental Handicap: Facilitating Holistic Care.* Sevenoaks: Hodder and Stoughton.

Barton R (1950) *Institutional Neurosis.* Bristol: Wright and Sons.

Benner P (1984) *From Novice to Expert – Excellence and Power in Clinical Nursing Practice.* Menlo Park, CA: Addison-Wesley.

Carle N (1984) *Key Concepts in Community Based Services.* London: Campaign for Mental Handicap.

DHSS (1979) *Report of the Committee of Enquiry into Mental Handicap Nursing and Care.* (Jay report). London: HMSO.

DHSS (1988) *Community Care: Agenda for Action.* Report to the Secretary of State for Social Services (Griffiths report). London: HMSO.

George J (1985) *Nursing Theories: The Base for Professional Practice.* Englewood Cliffs, NJ: Prentice Hall.

Grunewald K (1972) The guiding environment: the dynamics of residential living. In Boswell D & Wingrove, J, eds, *The Handicapped Person in the Community.* London: Tavistock Publications with the Open University.

Gunzburg H (1970) The hospital as a normalising training environment. *Journal of Mental Subnormality,* **16,** 71–83.

Henderson V (1966) *The Nature of Nursing.* London: Collier Macmillan.

Johnson D (1980) The behavioural system model for nursing. In Riehl J & Roy C, eds, *Conceptual Models for Nursing Practice.* Norwalk, CT: Appleton Century Crofts.

King I (1971) *Toward a Theory of Nursing.* New York: Wiley.

Maslow A (1943) A theory of human motivation. *Psychological Review,* **50,** 370–396.

Neuman B (1974) The Betty Neuman health care systems model: A total approach to patient problems. In Riehl J & Roy C eds, *Conceptual Models for Nursing Practice.* Norwalk, CT: Appleton Century Crofts.

O'Brien J (1981) *The Principle of Normalisation: A Foundation for Effective Services* (adapted by Tyne A.). London: Campaign for Mentally Handicapped People.

Orem D (1971) *Nursing: Concepts of Practice.* New York: McGraw-Hill.

Pearson A & Vaughan B (1986) *Nursing Models for Practice.* London: Heinemann.

Peplau H (1952) *Interpersonal Relations in Nursing.* New York: Pitman.

Rogers M (1970) *An Introduction to the Theoretical Basis of Nursing.* Philadelphia: Davis.

Roper N, Logan W and Tierney A (1980) *The Elements of Nursing.* Edinburgh: Churchill Livingstone.

Roy C (1984) *Introduction to Nursing: An Adaptation Model*, 2nd edn. Englewood Cliffs, NJ: Prentice Hall.

World Health Organisation (1961) *Constitution of WHO.* Basic Document, 15th edn. Geneva: WHO.

Wolfensberger W (1972) *Normalisation: The Principle of Normalisation in Human Services.* National Institute on Mental Retardation, Canada.

Wright S (1986) *Building and Using a Model of Nursing.* London: Edward Arnold.

Young W (1987) *Introduction to Nursing Concepts.* California: Appleton and Large.

Models for Nursing 2
Edited by B Kershaw and J Salvage
© 1990 Scutari Press

10

A Planned Approach to Nursing Children

ALAN GLASPER

Paediatric nurses have a long history of endeavouring to improve the care of their patients and families. The child and family are now viewed as an indivisible unit, and planning care for a sick child intimately involves the parents or guardians. The concept of a Care by Parent Unit has accentuated this philosophy (Sainsbury 1986); parents actively participate in their children's care under the guidance of trained children's nurses. With correct tuition parents are able to carry out specialist nursing tasks, and in some instances take over care completely.

The paediatric unit at Southampton, once a children's hospital in its own right, now occupies a floor of a large district general teaching hospital. It is fortunate enough to have a university department of child health close by. It consists of five distinct clinical areas, plus a large, thriving day unit catering primarily for children requiring surgery and maintenance oncology treatment.

Children who were once in hospital for long periods are now discharged into the care of the primary health team as quickly as possible. Southampton has an excellent cohort of paediatric community nurses, and tertiary care is kept to the minimum.

Like many other British units, however, Southampton has experienced some difficulty in introducing the nursing process and individualised nursing care. One of the main problems is that the time spent on individualised care plans, sometimes retrospectively, has been given a lower priority than the delivery of care, a dilemma not unique to paediatric nursing (Glasper, Stonehouse & Martin 1987). Although committed to the philosophy of individualised care, the unit's senior nurses established that there was a relationship between reduced staff numbers and an increase in admissions, with a corresponding decrease in the production of individualised care plans. The unit relies heavily on nursing students, often in their first year, to care for sick children and their families – but it is a myth that babies and children require only rudimentary nursing care (Glasper & Ireland 1988). Some staff have unrealistic expectations of first-level learners.

Conceptual models of nursing are becoming increasingly popular, but no one model has been designated for use exclusively in a paediatric setting, although several workers are experimenting with adaptations of existing ones (Glasper 1986, Casey 1988, Cheetham 1988). The four steps of the process of nursing can only be facilitated when a nurse has a cognitive tool at her disposal. Planning care in the absence of a conceptual framework is nursing in the dark. In times of stress and heavy workloads most nurses fall back on the traditional reactive medical model, which is perceived to be safe and practical; although in no way ideal, at least it is familiar to all.

Nursing students in Southampton learn about a full range of conceptual models, but the framework preferred in the health authority is based on an activities of living model. The preprinted assessment sheet used in the whole district is likewise based on an AL model, and the paediatric unit has a specially designed assessment sheet, also based on an AL model. In practice many care plans did not reflect the conceptual framework of the preprinted nursing process documents, but adhered to the traditional medical model.

The first task facing the paediatric unit was to make a conscious choice of nursing model. The nursing staff who had some acquaintance with the activity of living approach to nursing opted for the original Henderson framework (1966) rather than the anglicised Roper, Tierney and Logan adaptation (1980). Although not a model in the true sense of the word, the conceptual framework of Henderson was one the nurses felt comfortable with, while many accept that it is far from perfect. However, the nurses have an open mind about future developments in the choice of an appropriate model.

Most members of the team were familiar with Henderson's philosophy, but they had some difficulty in translating clinical nursing practice into appropriate terminology. There was, however, a mandate for adhering to the existing district documentation based on activities of living. Cost constraints prohibited the sea change that would have been required had another model been adopted. The use of nursing models may be considered in an evolutionary light; it may be necessary to begin with a simple model in order to make progress and to avoid the legacy of the past in imposing established models that colleagues feel are unsuitable.

Henderson's conceptual framework

Virginia Henderson is one of the greatest figures in nursing today, and her work is internationally acclaimed. Her interest in nursing developed during World War I and she graduated from the Army School of Nursing, Washington DC, in 1921. She became disillusioned during her training, when she came to see nursing as simply an extension of medicine. An impersonal approach was advocated and tuition was little more than watered-down instruction given to medical students. Only during her paediatric experience did she see the concept of patient-centred care in action and then, sadly, in the absence of the family. She realised the irony of the mechanistic medical model during her community experience, when she saw patients discharged from hospital into the same environment that had precipitated their original illness. Thus at an early stage she gave considerable thought to health education and the prevention of ill health.

After her graduation, Henderson chose to practise in a community setting. She eventually taught at Columbia Teachers College for nearly 20 years and put many of her ideas into practice. In 1955 she published her definition of nursing, modified in 1966 and still regarded as an outstanding contribution to nursing (Henderson 1966):

> 'The unique function of the nurse is to assist the individual, sick or well, in the performance of those activities contributing to health or its recovery (or to peaceful death) that he would perform unaided had he the necessary strength, will, or knowledge and to do this in such a way as to help him gain independence as rapidly as possible.'

Within this defined area Henderson believes the nurse to be the expert, the initiator and controller of her own activities. She recognises, however, that the nurse is part of a multidisciplinary team and as a consequence her work includes helping patients (families) carry out the physician's therapeutic plan.

The nurse, according to Henderson, is the substitute for what the patient (family) lacks to make him 'whole', 'complete' or 'independent' with respect to physical strength, will or knowledge:

> 'The nurse is temporarily the consciousness of the unconscious, the love of life for the suicide, the leg of the amputee, the eyes of the newly blind, a means of locomotion for the infant, knowledge and confidence for the young mother, a "voice" for those too weak or withdrawn to speak.'

It is thus the primary responsibility of the nurse to help the patient (family) with his daily pattern of living or with those activities he normally performs without assistance. Henderson elicits those activities as 14 basic needs, which in turn are seen as the 14 key components of basic nursing. These activities, with the definition above, are the heart of her conceptual framework:

1. Breathe normally.
2. Eat and drink adequately.
3. Eliminate body wastes.
4. Move and maintain desirable posture.
5. Sleep and rest.
6. Select suitable clothing – dress and undress.
7. Maintain body temperature within normal range by adjusting clothing and modifying the environment.
8. Keep the body clean and well groomed and protect the integument.
9. Avoid dangers in the environment and avoid injuring others.
10. Communicate with others in expressing emotions, needs, fears and opinions.
11. Worship according to one's faith.
12. Work in such a way that there is a sense of accomplishment.
13. Play or participate in various forms of recreation.

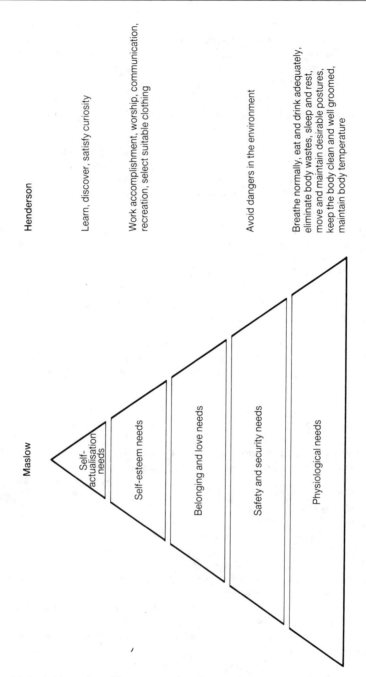

Figure. 10.1   A hierarchy of human needs (after Maslow 1943) and its relationship to Henderson's activities of living

14. Learn, discover, or satisfy the curiosity that leads to normal development and health and use of the available health facilities.

Henderson stresses that nursing is helping *with* and deciding *with*, not doing *for* and deciding *for*, except in certain circumstances such as coma, and helping in such a way as to encourage independence as soon as possible. In this way her conceptual framework is probably the precursor of the self-care model developed later by Dorothea Orem (Orem 1980).

Behavioural models of nursing which assume that people function in society by their own efforts owe much to Abraham Maslow's human needs theory (Maslow 1943). He regarded human responses to need as an integrated behavioural unit, emphasising the relationship between the various needs (Figure 10.1). The pyramidal nature of the hierarchy of needs shows physiological and safety needs as of paramount importance. Physiological needs must be met before progress at the next level of needs. Bluntly, survival is more important than the need for self-esteem. Likewise, according to Maslow it is useless to become self-actualised if one is unable to provide sustenance for oneself. There is little evidence to justify Maslow's rather simplistic view of human behaviour, but it remains an interesting concept.

In Henderson's activities of daily living, much of the focus is on the physiological and safety plane, with much less emphasis on Maslow's other areas of need. Henderson was deeply impressed by the concept of homeostasis and implied that the nurse must appreciate the concept of physiological balance. She sees the mind as inseparable from the body; thus physiological imbalance will affect emotional balance. Although she based many of her ideas on a concept of human needs, both physical and emotional, people's holistic nature does not seem to emerge. For example, the fact that a person's nutritional needs will have an effect on the other components of care is not made clear. If priority according to individual needs is implied in the list of ALs, is the presenting emotional problem given less emphasis than physical care? The fact that the 14 needs are focused primarily in the lower echelons of Maslow's hierarchy gives the impression that nursing care considerations are placed likewise. However, she does specify that the nurse must consider factors such as temperament and social and cultural status when assessing and prioritising patient care (Figure 10.1).

Henderson's philosophy was formulated many years before the nursing process. In many ways her work was a precursor of modern planned nursing care. She argued for individualised plans of care documented in a written format. Nursing action is deliberate, proactive and reactive, planned, executed and evaluated, and each of the 14 components must be assessed and prioritised. Only thus can the nurse identify problem areas, plan appropriate action and evaluate the outcomes. The involvement of the patient (family) at each step is fundamental to the planning of care. The patient actively participates in the care and the nurse carried out activities only when the patient is unable to carry them out for himself. Henderson stresses that the nurse must encourage the patient to be independent through the performance of the 14 basic components. Thus the planned nature of nursing, actively coupled with the emphasis on evaluation and written documentation, lends itself to the later development of the nursing process.

Using Henderson's framework in a paediatric setting

The ultimate justification for any conceptual nursing framework is its usefulness to client care. It must, of course, be relevant to the reality of nursing practice (Martin & Glasper 1986). Having decided to use Henderson's framework, the nurses' major task was to translate it into practice. It was decided to number each of Henderson's activities of daily living from 1 to 14. The abbreviated 'Henderson's needs identified' (HNI) followed by the specific index 1 to 14 was suggested as a method of relating patient problems to the activities of daily living. A further abbreviation PPA (patient problems arising) was suggested as a method of highlighting individual patient/family problems occurring with a specific need. All this proved satisfactory in that it enabled the reader of any care plan to identify with the conceptual framework and thus the method of problem-solving.

The greatest difficulty experienced was 'thinking' nursing and identifying patient problems in nursing terms. Initially, translating essentially medically-orientated problems to a nursing perspective using nursing terminology was crude, but it became increasingly sophisticated. In a first draft of a postoperative core care plan, 'potential nausea following anaesthetic' was substituted for 'problems with excretion'.

In most clinical areas the care plans are kept in a big plastic folder, one for each bay or cubicle. The largest bays have six beds and there may be up to six plans in one folder at any given time. A copy of Henderson's conceptual framework (Figure 10.2) is inserted in every folder, which proved popular and reinforced the adopted method.

Heavy workloads, however, caused much difficulty in adopting the chosen framework. The holistic philosophy of paediatric nursing is often at odds with reality in an acute clinical area with diminishing staff numbers. The reliance on

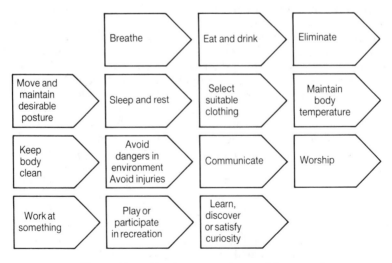

Figure 10.2   Henderson's conceptual framework

students exacerbates the problem. For many staff, putting this philosophy into practice seemed an impossible challenge. During busy periods the ability to support learners in the formulation of care plans was compromised, and resulted in plans that were incomplete, inadequate or out of date, or in a failure to produce any plans at all. In many instances plans were written 48–72 hours after admission, by which time many of the initial, potential or actual problems had changed. The use of the nursing process in the preparation of individualised plans came to be seen as an expensive and wasteful exercise which benefited no-one. The perceived failure of the plans to influence the quality of care meant that many staff saw no need to read them.

These difficulties reinforced existing problems in the use of written individual care plans. Experienced paediatric nurses failed to see the need for them when they had nursed numerous children with similar conditions in the past. Faced with the option of providing care or spending time writing plans they naturally chose the former. With little empirical evidence to support the view that individual written care plans resulted in better care, radical remedial action was required: the development and use of predetermined core nursing plans. Such plans had been successfully adopted by the hospital's adult medical unit, and it was agreed to conduct a limited experiment on one of the paediatric wards.

Designing core nursing plans

The impetus to design the plans therefore emerged from a conflict between the philosophy of the nursing process and the realities of ward workloads. The development of such plans is only possible when there is agreement between colleagues about the nursing management of particular child/family problems/needs. From this evolves a plan for a modicum of prescribed care commensurate with agreed standards of patient safety, for a period of not more than 72 hours. A specific conceptual nursing framework must be used to underpin the development of such plans, to avoid the pitfalls of prescribing care that is purely reactive to the medical diagnosis.

The staff were asked to ascertain from their ward records the incidence of certain types of conditions, from which a list was drawn up of the commonest causes of admission. The next step was to involve nurses in the preparation of ideal universal care plans where time was not a factor. Staff who volunteered were given simple instructions involving preparing a nursing care plan that included only the care they thought essential during the first 48–72 hours. The results were revealing: the plans they produced were extremely elaborate and represented what they would wish to see in a personalised plan had they the time. Using Henderson's conceptual framework they produced plans that were immensely long and could not possibly have been written in an acute clinical situation. It was, however, interesting to note that given time practitioners could produce high-quality plans.

The initial plans were then considered by a group of nurses who agreed to concentrate only on those child/family problems for which there was a high level of agreement regarding nursing interventions for a maximum of 72 hours after admission. Wright (1987) says that it is possible to use prewritten plans without stifling creativity; the production of our core nursing plans did indeed help the introduction of planned personalised care, and removed a major grievance concerning repetitive written statements. A number of predetermined plans were produced and their use in clinical practice is the subject of ongoing evaluation.

Having agreed the format of the plans, the staff of an acute surgical/trauma ward for children aged 4–16 years began to use them. They are printed on standard district care plan stationery and follow the Henderson framework outlined earlier. The design enables easy addition of handwritten, personalised entries. They are stored according to subject in a small filing cabinet near the nursing station, and are subject to the following guidelines:

1   It is the responsibility of the admitting nurse to ensure that the child has a current, valid care plan.

2   All predetermined core nursing plans must be individualised.

3   All care plans must be dated and signed, using a full signature.

4   Each problem area should be carefully considered as to its appropriateness, and ticked and signed for accordingly.

5   It may be necessary to post-date certain problems on the predetermined core nursing plans which are not current at any one particular period of time.

6   Predetermined core nursing plans do not have to be countersigned (all additions and handwritten care plans must be countersigned by a trained nurse).

7   All current patient problems should be evaluated on the care plan evaluation form at the end of the morning shift and when changes occur. Brief report from night staff.

Predetermined core nursing plans must be constructed by clinical nurse specialists such as ward sisters and staff nurses. Using Henderson's framework, only those activities of daily living usually compromised by a particular problem and of high priority are identified. There must be space on the printed plans to add extra problems, goals and interventions depending on individual circumstances. They have four main advantages in paediatric nursing practice. They enable paediatric nurses to escape from the burden of too much paperwork, especially in fast-changing circumstances; they provide a means of identifying the crucial immediate care required by sick children within a conceptual framework of nursing; they are a means of helping staff explain rationales of care to juniors; and they facilitate quality assurance, as most methods of nursing audit rely on evaluating documentation.

Sarah: a case study

Sarah Wilkins, aged 12 years, was admitted to a paediatric surgical unit for correction of an idiopathic scoliosis. Her spinal abnormality was detected six months previously during a routine school medical examination. Her mother had noticed that the hem of her daughter's uniform skirt was not hanging properly, but attributed this to Sarah's dislike of the uniform. After the initial diagnosis the scoliosis appeared to worsen and this was confirmed after a subsequent X-ray. The orthopaedic surgeon decided to advise operative intervention after discussion with Sarah and her family.

On admission, data were collected from Sarah and her parents and a plan of care (Figure 10.3) was initiated. A predetermined core nursing plan based on Henderson's activities of living was initiated and personalised to cater for Sarah and her family's needs. The plan was designed by the staff of the unit to address only those commonalities of care shared by all children admitted for correction of scoliosis. The subsequent personalisation of the plan was carried out only after a full audit of the family's needs by the admitting nurse. This process is mandatory in the formation of a personal, workable plan. All problems, actual and potential, are evaluated by the team leaders at the end of every shift (or more often as necessary). An evaluation sheet, which accompanies the plan, helps to ensure that current problems are fully evaluated.

On initial contact the admitting nurse soon ascertained the family's anxiety: Sarah herself freely admitted she was 'scared to death'. Using Henderson's framework and in consideration of the need to communicate, the predetermined care plan identifies anxiety as a major problem in the preoperative phase. It suggests specific standards of care which should be met to ensure resolution of the problem. The plan allows for personalisation and in the example given the nurse has prescribed the use of a Zaadie doll, one of a new generation of anatomical models developed specifically for children in hospital. They are cloth-covered and have three layers which peel apart using velcro fastenings to expose their vital organs; a simple yet effective design.

The paediatric unit is planning a preadmission programme for children and their families. Psychological preparation can then be given in advance: preparing children for fear-evoking events has been shown to be effective in clinical practice (Rodin 1983). In the absence of such a programme at the time of Sarah's admission, other strategies had to be employed.

Many adults use inappropriate language when explaining aspects of treatment to children. This is especially true of hospital staff, who are often confronted with an infinite variety of explanations of illness. What may be appropriate for a 12-year-old may be wholly inappropriate for a four-year-old. Child health workers should be able to offer a variety of treatment explanations consistent with the child's cognitive development. In the case of Sarah and her parents, the nurse decided to address their specific fears by ascertaining their level of anatomical understanding, and augmenting it through the use of the Zaadie doll. The nurse and play therapist explained the operation using the doll and X-ray films. As Sarah was going to be catheterised during surgery and would remain so for several days, a demonstration of the procedure was conducted on the doll. She found this therapeutic play most beneficial and many of her hidden fears were explored: she had been particularly concerned about how she would 'go to the toilet' while lying on the spinal bed. The plan of care addressed this topic and the nurse let Sarah and her parents investigate the Stryker frame. Sarah was encouraged to lie on the bed and be turned several times. The plan also recommended that Sarah be introduced to other children with similar conditions; fortunately she was able to meet another girl of similar age recovering from a spinal fusion operation performed the previous week. The nurse left Sarah and her

HNI = Henderson's need identified
PPA = Patient problems arising

1. Breathe.   2. Eat and drink.   3. Eliminate.   4. Move and maintain desirable posture.   5. Sleep and rest.
6. Select suitable clothing.   7. Maintain body temperature.   8. Keep body clean.
9. Avoid dangers in environment/avoid injuries.   10. Communicate.   11. Worship.   12. Work at something.
13. Play or participate in recreation.

Problem/need	Goal	Action to be taken
1 HNI 10 PPA		
(a) Child/parental anxiety regarding impending surgery/anaesthesia	Facilitate full and frank discussion	Explain all procedures specific to the child's surgery Use appropriate models/X-rays to explain where required Introduce to other families who have had similar experiences Introduce Sarah to Zaadie dolls
(b) Lack of familiarity with ward	Orientate family to ward/ and school	Show around the ward Introduce to Mary, the school teacher Explain any ward routines Offer parental accommodation as required Explain meal times, etc. Allow Sarah to eat with parents in dining room
(c) Apprehension related to being nursed on a Stryker frame	Fully orientate child to the Stryker frame	Prepare Stryker frame with clean linen Check all mechanical parts Allow child and family to witness nursing staff using the frame Let parents experience turns Allow child to play/investigate frame before encouraging a practice turn Introduce to other children being nursed on a Stryker frame Allow child to sleep on frame prior to surgery if desired Explain how child will pass urine/open bowels while on frame Obtain full and detailed nursing history
2 HNI 9 PPA		
Correct identification of operation site	Assist surgeon with the insertion of the spinal marker	Ensure aseptic technique used throughout Explain procedure to child Place child in position as for lumbar puncture Allow parental presence where desired Child may resume normal activities after procedure

Figure 10.3 Predetermined care plan for a child having posterior spinal fusion for scoliosis

Problem/need	Goal	Action to be taken
3 HNI 2 PPA Potential asphyxia or delay in surgery caused by accidental oral intake immediately before surgery/anaesthesia	Remain nil orally as per instructions	Ascertain time of nil-by-mouth (2 a.m.) Offer last drink as instructed (at least 6 hours before surgery); may have late supper Explain to parents and child the reason for this Place nil-by-mouth notice on bedhead Remove all fluids, sweets, fruit, etc. from child's locker Observe younger age groups carefully for non-compliance
4 HNI 3 PPA Potential contamination of wound caused by bowel action during surgery	Prevent contamination of operation site	Ensure child voids urine before surgery (immediately before premedication if possible) Ascertain time of last bowel action Bowel prep where indicated
5 HNI 8 PPA Potential wound contamination caused by inadequate skin preparation	Ensure child arrives in theatre clean	Preoperative bath – check nails and hair Observe and report any abnormalities Dress child in operative clothing after bath and before transfer
6 HNI 9 PPA Potential operative/postoperative complications	Ensure safe surgery/anaesthesia	Ensure identification bands in position and checked Ensure consent form signed Remove any prosthesis, cosmetics or jewellery Check and record any allergies Record weight Check contact with infectious disease Report any deviation of vital signs or indications of respiratory infection Administer prescribed premedication Confine patient to bed after premedication Place cot sides in position where indicated Ensure that theatre checklist is completed Apply local anaesthetic cream to dorsum of left hand

Figure 10.3   Predetermined care plan for a child having posterior spinal fusion for scoliosis, continued

parents with Janet for half an hour. During this time Janet had to be turned as part of her regular schedule. Sarah greatly appreciated watching this, especially as Janet reported that the only bad thing about the Stryker frame was boredom.

Sarah was a little shocked to see her friend wheeled off down the corridor some time later. The nurse informed her that Janet was going to school. At this point, and as previously indicated on the plan, the nurse suggested that Sarah might like to meet the teachers. Sarah had not considered school as part of being in hospital.

Although the plan suggested that Sarah might like to sleep on the Stryker frame during the first night in hospital, this was declined; she said she would rather sleep in a normal bed until her operation. The plan had catered for parental accommodation and this was duly offered to her mother, who wanted to stay with Sarah for the first two preoperative nights. It had been explained that Sarah would spend the subsequent three nights in a high care area adjacent to the nurses' station.

The following day, as indicated on the plan under the need to maintain a safe environment, the senior house officer and the nurse discussed with Sarah and her family the need to insert a spinal marker. Sarah was naturally worried by the procedure; she was shown Janet's X-rays, which clearly highlighted the spinal marker. After reassurance about the effectiveness of the local anaesthetic she accompanied the nurse and the house officer to the treatment room. Sarah's father was willing to stay and help with the procedure but her mother declined. After the procedure Sarah proudly told her mother, 'It didn't hurt a bit'.

On the morning of surgery the need to eat and drink were highlighted on the predetermined plan as one of a series of compromised needs necessitated by impending anaesthesia and surgery. This aspect of the plan was commensurate with the standard criteria for the safe reception of a child in theatre.

A predetermined postoperative core care plan likewise facilitated successful nursing interventions after surgery, until personalised care based on the child's own needs was established.

The use of Henderson's conceptual framework in clinical practice is well documented and encourages an easy if somewhat pragmatic approach to nursing care. The advent of family-centred care in many paediatric units is making the limitations of this type of model more apparent. For the moment care plans based on activities of living offer paediatric practitioners a reliable solution to some of the problems they face.

References

Casey A (1988) A partnership with child and family. *Senior Nurse,* **8**(4), 8–9.

Cheetham T (1988) Model care in the surgical ward. *Senior Nurse,* **8**(4), 10–12.

Glasper E (1986) Scaling down a model. *Nursing Times,* **82**(43), 57–58.

Glasper E & Ireland L (1988) A special kind of learner, *Senior Nurse,* **8**(4), April.

Glasper E, Stonehouse J & Martin L (1987) Core care plans. *Nursing Times,* **83**(10), 55–57.

Henderson V (1966) *The Nature of Nursing.* London: Collier Macmillan.

Martin L & Glasper E (1986) Core plans – nursing models and the nursing process in action. *Nursing Practice,* **1**(4), 268–273.

Maslow A (1943) A theory of human motivation. *Psychological Review*, **50,** 370–396.

Orem D (1980) *Nursing: Concepts of Practice*. New York: McGraw-Hill.

Rodin J (1983) *Will This Hurt?* London: Royal College of Nursing.

Roper N, Logan W & Tierney A (1980) *The Elements of Nursing*. Edinburgh: Churchill Livingstone.

Sainsbury C (1986) Care by parents of their children in hospital. *Archives of Disease in Childhood*, **61,** 612–615.

Wright S (1987) Producing practical care plans. *Nursing Times*, **83**(38), 24–27.

Models for Nursing 2
Edited by B Kershaw and J Salvage
© 1990 Scutari Press

11

Knowing That and Knowing How: The Role of the Lecturer Practitioner

BARBARA VAUGHAN

The challenge that faces nurses today may be the greatest and most significant since the Nightingale era. New ideas are being generated in an attempt to clarify the purpose of nursing itself and hence the service that nurses offer patients/ clients. Furthermore, views of health care are under question, with a shift in emphasis from the traditional biomedical model of care to the more holistic approach inherent in most models of nursing. Patients, who have been largely acquiescent in the past, are becoming more knowledgeable about their own health and recognising the rights they have for choice, information and public accountability.

The changes being advocated in nursing require much more than a theoretical understanding of nursing models or the nursing process, however. Fundamental shifts are needed in attitudes towards practice and the way in which nursing work is managed if progress is to be made. For example, there is no way in which the personalised care or therapeutic relationships advocated in many models can be introduced to their full extent unless there are changes in the structure in which nursing takes place, with each nurse being given the room and freedom to work as a professional practitioner. Moreover, unless the nurses concerned are prepared to accept the responsibility and hence accountability that is part of professional practice, progress will inevitably be limited. Learning to practise in a way that differs significantly from traditional approaches is no easy matter. The interrelationship of the factors that have to be considered is complex, and mistakes may be made if the complexity of the situation is not recognised.

Knowing that and knowing how

In thinking about how the use of a nursing model can be beneficial to nurses, and more importantly to clients, we must remember that it is relatively easy to learn something new from a theoretical perspective, but much more difficult to put that new learning into practice. Thus it is not uncommon for nurses to hear of one set of ideas and values that are taught in theory but to see another set of values used in practice. Furthermore, there is some evidence that even in those areas which profess to have adopted a nursing model as their framework for practice the change is only skin deep and, while lip service is paid to a new approach, in reality no changes have occurred and old ways are perpetuated (Kapelli 1986). Thus there are nurses who 'know' about models of nursing from a textbook perspective and advocate this approach to practice, but understandably have much greater difficulty in 'doing' in practice. There is consequently a mismatch between the two, with a gap between what is advocated and what actually happens. Yet in a practice discipline such as nursing the most valuable contributors to the service must be the 'knowledgeable doers', those who not only know 'that' but also know 'how'.

It is not difficult to see how this situation has arisen. The manner in which nursing has developed has led to clear distinctions between those who have remained in practice, those who have moved into nurse education, those who have advanced their careers in nurse management and those who have become researchers. A false division has grown, with different branches advancing at different rates and sometimes in different directions. A major barrier against giving any one person legitimate authority over more than one aspect of nursing work has been created; the clinician has little say in the field of education and the person who holds a formal role in education has no right to lead practice.

This division has inevitably led to difficulties in the development of practice, such as the introduction of a nursing model, since there is no single named person who can take nursing forward as a whole and influence both practice and education. Situations arise were there is a mismatch between what is done and what is taught. If the development and use of nursing models is to be encouraged, and there are many who would strongly support this, three major areas must be considered which have, to some extent, been ignored in the past.

Firstly, there is the knowledge required for practice. Trying to introduce new ways without giving people the opportunity to learn can be seen as a recipe for disaster. Any nursing model contains a clear indication of the knowledge seen as essential for advanced practice, and in some instances this has been used as the basis for preregistration curriculum design. However, there is evidence that the opportunity for experienced nurses to update their knowledge along the same lines is scanty, with wide national variation (Rogers & Lawrence 1987). Furthermore it can be suggested that the help needed goes far beyond formal learning to realistic consideration of the implications for practice and how that knowledge may be put to use.

Secondly, there is a major area to consider concerned with knowledge of self. Unless nurses perceive themselves as professional practitioners, contributing on an equal footing with other health care workers and willing to accept the consequences of their actions, their contribution is much less likely to be effective. There may be gender issues giving rise to the apparent lack of value nurses place on their own work. From a societal point of view nursing is still seen as subservient to medicine, a view to some extent perpetuated by nurses themselves.

Orlando (1987) argues that many nurses have chosen the path of role extension, the acceptance of tasks traditionally undertaken by doctors, and place higher value on this type of work than in the development of nursing as an independent but complementary discipline. Yet a brief overview of the literature related to nursing models will clearly identify areas of client need that nurses could or should expand their role to meet, provided they recognise fully the value of this contribution and are prepared to stand accountable for their part in the total health care service.

Finally, consideration has to be given to the manner in which nursing work is organised. Implicit in many of the nursing models is an understanding that nursing is offered by independent practitioners who have the freedom to manage their own work, rather than being hidebound by the rules and regulations of a rigid hierarchy. Yet in reality many nurses are still caught in a management system and structure that gives them little room to practise in this way. The evidence of Strong and Robinson (1988) suggests that nurses are still hanging on to traditional models of organisation which allow strict control, even though there is an expectation of personalised care for patients. Many senior practitioners are still unable to appoint their own staff; they are constrained within off-duty patterns that are arranged centrally rather than to meet the needs of their client group; they are expected to comply with some rules in relationship to practice that have been defined by others; or they are expected to follow a philosophy of care that has been decreed centrally rather than agreed at clinical level.

A way forward

Many of the changes in nursing have taken an approach where attempts were made to change one small part of the total system, such as the introduction of care plans, without thought being given to the content of the plans, the knowledge of those who would be preparing them, or the way in which they would be used. Thus a new system has been superimposed on an old one without looking at the effect of one small change on the whole picture. For example, in many areas in which care plans have been introduced nurses have continued to hold the traditional ward report, and then wonder why the care plans are not being used. In reality the same work is being undertaken in two different ways: care was being prescribed in the traditional manner during the ward report, so that many saw no point in using the care plans. What could have been a valuable asset to nursing became an extra chore, with its real purpose lost in the traditional ward style.

It would seem important to avoid a repetition with the introduction of nursing models. If full advantage is to be taken of their potential use to nursing, radical changes are required which take account of the total situation.

Although there is never a single right way of introducing new ideas to nursing, one approach to overcoming the difficulties experienced in the past is to consider the introduction of what have been called 'unified roles'; that is, roles where the authority and hence responsibility for all aspects of professional practice are vested in a single person. This does not mean that this person has to do everything herself, but that she has legitimate authority for practice, the management of a clinical unit, education and research. One role that moves along this path is that of the lecturer practitioner (Vaughan 1987). Ideas for the development of this role emerged from concern about the difficulties experienced by both practitioners and educators in finding a match between what was being done in practice and what was being taught in theory, as well as a fundamental belief in the value of practice as the origin of much nursing theory. The ideas were developed further with the acknowledgement that radical change is required in existing patterns of nurse education, reinforced by the government's acceptance of the Project 2000 recommendations (UKCC 1986). If the curricula of the future are to be developed around nursing models, the need to find a match between practice and education becomes even more urgent.

If changes are to be made, however, it is important that there is a sound rationale for moving from old ways. Thus we must examine how nursing has been developed in the past before making significant changes to a structure for the future, so that old lessons are not forgotten and note is taken of what is feasible.

Traditional roles in nursing

The issue of effective teaching of the practice of nursing has been examined for many years and several ways forward have been explored. Traditionally the responsibility for teaching practice was vested in the ward sister, but by the mid-1960s it was becoming apparent that this was impossible in the context of the increasing dependency of hospital patients and the increasing workload. The formal teaching of practice became the province of the nurse teacher, with the introduction of the role of clinical teacher, although more recently many tutors have undertaken this responsibility. Anyone who has been a clinical teacher knows that this is not an easy role to fulfil and requires skilled teaching. It is also interesting to note that when this role was first introduced the qualifications to teach the practice of nursing were less rigorous than those required to teach the theory, which says something about the relative value placed on the two areas in reality. Integrating theory in a turbulent and unpredictable environment is in many ways more difficult than teaching in the relatively safe classroom environment.

In theory the idea of clinical teaching may have appeared sensible but the reality was far from satisfactory; several arguments highlight the difficulties experienced. Part of the responsibility of the clinical teacher was to ensure that the environment in which the student was working was conducive to her learning needs and complementary to the theoretical teaching. However, since the teacher had no control over what was taught in theory or what was done in practice, the task was almost impossible. For instance, if the framework for practice used in the educational programme followed the ideas of Orem (1980) but the nurses in practice were using an alternative model, there would inevitably be a mismatch.

The leadership of the clinical team is vested in the ward sister/charge nurse, and rightly so. But in practice this means that everyone else who enters the environment is, in essence, a visitor to her domain, including the teacher, who has no actual authority for practice. No problems arise if there is no discrepancy between what has been taught and what is happening, but this is often not the case. For example, in teaching about pain management the use of pain assessment tools and techniques such as massage and distraction may have been introduced. The teacher has no authority to ensure that these methods are also considered in practice, nor can she guarantee that the team leader will be interested in introducing them. She is entirely dependent on negotiation from a very weak stance.

As an intermittent visitor to the ward, the teacher may also have difficulty in maintaining her clinical competence. In Benner's view (1984) the expert practitioner is someone who has gained an understanding of clients' nursing needs through in-depth study and knowledge of the particular clinical setting. This can only be gained over a period of time, so that the nurse can become sensitive to the cues of what is happening around her, and in Benner's view it can take up to five years. Furthermore, this ability is not directly transferable; an expert in one area cannot immediately become an expert elsewhere, but needs time to recognise the cues in the new environment.

If Benner's criteria are accepted, the difficulties of intermittent clinical teaching become even more evident. There is a possible loss of credibility in the eyes of the student if what is advocated in theory is not witnessed in practice. Furthermore, some teachers find it hard to accept the reality of practice or acknowledge the need for priority-setting. This may be understandable, since their prime responsibility is helping students to learn, but it does not help students to face the reality of the work situation. As Kramer (1974) pointed out, this was one of the factors that caused the greatest conflict for students and contributed to the high attrition rate. In parallel with this, there are sisters who are not up to date in their thinking about practice, so conflict inevitably arises.

Some of the difficulties identified so far can be overcome and many teachers and sisters have achieved good results in these difficult circumstances. However, fundamental issues have arisen more recently which serve to increase the difficulties. The importance of the relationship between the client and the care-giver is recognised in many nursing models, but it cannot be developed through intermittent visits to the clinical unit. The continuity itself is fundamental to primary nursing, or indeed any form of professional practice, but if it is only possible to visit the unit intermittently the possibility of demonstrating this skill as a role model – a very powerful mode of teaching – is limited. The intermittent visits could also be seen as disruptive to the therapeutic programme established with the patient.

A further issue that challenges the role of the clinical teacher is the need for any professional practitioner to be able to relate the 'actions of today' to the 'outcomes of tomorrow'. In other words, there is a need to relate the process of nursing to the outcomes for the patients if we are to gather data to help us understand how nursing may help patients. Teachers may be in a good position to debate these topics, but unless they can see for themselves the effects of planned nursing interventions in the long term as well as the short term, it is difficult for them to evaluate their usefulness and increase their understanding of nursing. The question has to be raised of whether this is the most effective and efficient way of teaching the practice of nursing.

Joint appointees

One of the ways people have tried to overcome some of these difficulties has been the creation of joint appointees, that is nurses with a foot in both camps; many people who fulfil these roles have been very successful. But we must ask whether this is a role the majority would be prepared to undertake. Two roles have been superimposed, one on top of another, without consideration of which parts of the role can be discarded. In many cases this results in an expectation that all aspects of both roles will be fulfilled, requiring some sort of Superman to be able to function effectively. While there is little doubt that the sentiment behind the creation of these roles was worthy, the reality of practice was another story.

A new approach

With the growing recognition of the value of using a nursing model in practice, and the rapid changes in nursing education, the time is ripe to consider alternative ways of developing. Furthermore, while the authority for teaching the theory and practice of nursing remains vested in separate people, the dissonance created by a variance between what is taught and what is done could become even more exaggerated and the so-called theory–practice gap could widen. Nor will it be feasible to develop the science and the art of nursing effectively if we perpetuate the difference between taught and used theory. Clinical teaching has failed to overcome the problem and, although joint appointments have gone some way towards resolving it, the role is fraught with its own problems of shared leadership, lack of continuity, role conflict, role overload and role confusion. With these thoughts in mind, a new approach to the creation of a unified role is suggested here.

If unified roles are to be developed in nursing they have to be considered in the context of the whole structure of practice and education, rather than as an adjunct to the present system. Thus we must consider how clinical work is managed, the management system of the organisation as a whole, and the educational system.

Relating what has happened in the past to social policy, it would seem that the creation of clinical teaching was the classic first-level approach to change – splitting off a component of a job that seemed too big – with all the inherent difficulties already discussed. This was in fact the Salmon report's recommendation on the role of the ward sister, with the consequent removal of authority for housekeeping and providing food to patients (Ministry of Health 1966). Yet today, one of the commonest laments from clinical units is the sister's lack of control over these two aspects of work – maybe there is a lesson to be learned here!

Another common approach when considering new roles is to impose a new aspect of work on a traditional role without considering which aspects of the role can be shed. This is the experience of some joint appointees, with the difficulties outlined above. A third approach, which Vickers (1965) suggests may be the most successful but is also the most difficult, is to restructure the concepts that relate to the work to be achieved. This is what the unified role of the lecturer practitioner is all about.

The lecturer practitioner

Lecturer practitioners have responsibility and authority for both practice and education within a defined clinical area, with two broad but clearly defined aims:

1 to identify and maintain the standards of practice and policies within a defined clinical area;
2 to prepare and contribute to the educational programme of students in relation to the theory and practice of nursing in that unit.

While research is not defined as a separate area, there is an understanding that, as with any other professional practitioner, the responsibility for it would be incorporated in the role. Thus the nurse would be in a position to ensure that there is a match between the clinical and educational models in use. To be able to achieve these functions, lecturer practitioners also need to accept some managerial responsibility, since otherwise they could not control the clinical environment or create a setting conducive not only to client care but also to learning. Thus clinical/managerial responsiblities would include

● clarifying the ward philosophy, goals and framework for practice in conjuction with the rest of the clinical team, and ensuring that all staff understand and work towards them;
● acting in a consultancy role to the clinical staff in relationship to nursing practice;
● identifying the professional development needs of the unit staff and ensuring that they are met;
● carrying a small clinical caseload, either intermittently or continuously (this could be done in various ways according to the clinical specialty and the way work is organised);
● identifying the nursing policies of the unit and ensuring that they are followed;
● setting the standards of practice of the unit and ensuring that they are achieved;
● establishing and maintaining communication networks within and outside the unit.

The lecturer practitioner would also, as a consequence, require authority for managing the skill mix within the ward budget, and for making staff appointments and reviewing performance. There must be a significant flattening of the traditional hierarchy still prevalent in nursing and a move towards vesting authority in those responsible for the direct delivery of care. This does not mean that one person has to do all these things herself; some can appropriately be delegated to other team members once standards have been set. However, it does mean the lecturer practitioner has authority and hence control in unifying the functions.

The educational responsibilities would include:

● planning the educational experience of students in the unit, in conjuction with a course committee, to meet the specific learning objectives of the theory and practice of nursing as identified in the curriculum;

- organising the educational experience for the students in the clinical unit and contributing to the teaching;
- arranging assessments for the students, in conjunction with the examinations committee.

When there are no student placements the lecturer practitioner may contribute to teaching outside the unit; become involved with other educational activities such as curriculum development; and, most importantly, continue personal and professional development through further study and research.

By vesting in one person the authority for the policies of the unit, the professional development of the permanent staff and the student programme, it would be possible to ensure that each area of responsibility dovetailed with the next. Thus, if a particular model of nursing was taught in a formal setting, the manner in which it had been modified to suit the clinical unit, and the difficulties experienced in its use in practice, could be incorporated into the discussion. Furthermore, there would be an increased likelihood that the practitioners with whom the students worked would have a similar, hopefully deeper understanding of the practical use of the chosen approach. Thus 'self-care' or 'positive adaptation' would become more than an approach read about in a textbook – a working guide to practice.

The setting

The current clinical structure needs rethinking in order to facilitate the development of a role of this nature. The sister role, directly responsible and accountable for all the nursing prescribed and delivered in the ward, would no longer exist in teaching areas and would be replaced by the lecturer practitioner role. Introducing a system of primary nursing would devolve many of the functions of the traditional ward sister to those who deliver the care. If the primary nurse accepts responsibility for care planning for a named group of patients alongside the additional work of liaising with other health care workers, arranging discharge, linking with family members and so on, much of the sister's time is freed; and by introducing a secretarial post much of the time spent by many sisters on clerical and administrative (rather than managerial) work would also be freed.

Qualifications

This is a highly skilled role requiring expertise in clinical practice and education. As an absolute minimum level of preparation, it requires a Diploma in Nursing and an approved educational qualification; experience in ward management would also be required. These are only seen as a starting point and future demand will be much higher, but since the number of nurses with more advanced qualifications is limited it would be unrealistic to expect more. Similarly, if the system is to work the primary nurse must have sufficient knowledge and experience to be able to accept the responsibility of a personal caseload, so some evidence of study beyond the first level of qualification should be sought.

Organisation

In recent years there has been a trend towards minimal differentiation between the work of the sister and other registered nurses, counting heads rather than considering the work people should be doing in different roles. Indeed, it is not uncommon to hear the 'good' sister described as one who can roll up her sleeves and get on with the job. It has also become the norm for her presence to be essential for sufficient cover. Yet sometimes this is at the cost of other aspects of work, possibly less immediately enjoyable but nevertheless essential, such as forward planning, teaching, clarification of standards and staff appraisal. In this context it would be extremely difficult to make a formal move to introduce a model, since the work undertaken and the expectations of what is 'good' do not allow time for development.

Such expectations would have to alter if a role such as that of the lecturer practitioner is to succeed. Firstly, it would be necessary to exclude the lecturer practitioner from the establishment seen as essential to provide safe cover. This does not mean that she would not deliver clinical care from time to time, but this could be done through acting as an associate nurse, carrying a very small caseload or working intermittently as a primary nurse. The lecturer practitioner would have to be an expert in clinical practice in order to fulfil the consultancy function, however. Secondly, change is needed in the expectations that staff nurses and senior nurses have of the traditional sister, with recognition of the importance of all aspects of her work. There may be a need to be much more systematic about the relationship of the clinical workload to the staffing of a unit, with recognition that as patient dependency has increased over the years a mismatch has often developed between patients' needs and the nursing hours available to give care. This further emphasises the need for expert and experienced nurses to retain direct authority over practice, since only they can gather relevant data to present arguments for adequate nursing cover.

A further change that would help the development of this role is to reshape the way many senior nurses work. The traditional pattern in nursing has been a hierarchy of control, but in many instances what is required is a support system that provides a service to practitioners to facilitate their work. Many such services would ease the life of the practitioner, such as help with dependency work, through making available established systems or considering new ways; helping to introduce quality assurance methods which may identify areas for development rather than act as punitive measures; negotiating with other services to ensure that clinical nursing time is not wasted on looking for equipment or linen – the list could go on for ever. What is important is a shift in relationship from seniority to mutual respect and support. This is not an easy shift for many nurses, who have been used to a system of hierarchies, but it has to be considered if we wish to develop professional practitioners.

Feasibility

An immediate response to the description of this role has been that it is too big for one person. However, the suggestions put forward should be considered in the light of other recommendations which require considerable organisational and attitudinal change. For example, the introduction of primary nursing requires communication with other health care workers who have traditionally expected to 'see sister'; some tasks that have been seen as 'high value' may be redistributed to secretarial staff who have been prepared to undertake them; primary nurses who have been used to deferring all decisions to sister have to learn to work more independently. The movement towards such major changes may be long and hard, but experience suggests that they are feasible and worthwhile in the long run.

The role described here is one potential way of facilitating the development of model-based practice. Emphasis has been given to freeing space to incorporate a teaching function in the practice role traditionally known as the sister or charge nurse. However, it is equally feasible to consider developing the clinical role in other ways once time has been freed in the way suggested. For example, it may be appropriate for some practitioners to develop a more formal research function. Others may be particularly interested in developing skills related to the management of the total organisation, with a view to moving into general management. What is important is that the full implications of such changes are recognised and that imagination is used in trying to find a way forward.

Many of these points may seem distant from the idea of introducing models to nursing practice. Yet, returning to my initial argument, it can be suggested that while the authority for practice and education remains segregated in nursing, the dissonance that occurs through the variance between what is taught and what is done will not be overcome. Furthermore, there are many places where attempts to introduce changes to practice have been fraught with difficulty because the broader implications were not acknowledged. The clinician has frequently been hampered by organisational constraints such as inappropriate rules and regulations, fixed shift patterns, the inability to alter skill mixes to suit the developments, or unsuitable and sometimes outmoded teaching. Similarly, many teachers have been frustrated by their lack of ability to go further than talking about some of the valuable aspects of nursing models. The time may have come to be radical in our thinking; while the changes may be slow in being realised, we should plan for a major readjustment in the way nursing is organised in order to be able to enhance practice.

References

Benner P (1984) *From Novice to Expert – Excellence and Power in Clinical Nursing Practice.* Menlo Park, CA: Addison Wesley.
Kapelli S (1986) Nurses' management of patients' self care. *Nursing Times*, **82** (11), 40–43.
Kramer M (1974) *Reality Shock.* New York: C V Mosby.
Ministry of Health, Scottish and Home Health Department (1966) *Report of the Committee on Senior Nursing Staff Structure* (Salmon report). London: HMSO.
Orem D (1980) *Nursing: Concepts of Practice.* New York: McGraw-Hill.
Orlando I (1987) Nursing in the 21st century – alternative paths. *Journal of Advanced Nursing*, **12**(4), 405–412.

Rogers J & Lawrence J (1987) *Continuing Professional Education for Qualified Nurses, Midwives and Health Visitors*. Peterborough: Ashdale Press.

Strong P & Robinson J (1988) *New Model Management – Griffiths and the NHS*. Report No 3. University of Warwick: Nursing Policy Studies Centre.

UKCC (1986) *Project 2000: A New Preparation for Practice*. London: UKCC.

Vaughan B (1987) Bridging the gap – teaching roles in nurse education. *Senior Nurse*, **6**(5), 30–31.

Vickers G, ed. (1965) *The Art of Judgement*. London: Harper and Row.

Models for Nursing 2
Edited by B Kershaw and J Salvage
© 1990 Scutari Press

12

Conceptual Framework or Work Method? A Study of the Nursing Process in One School of Nursing

PAM SMITH

In this chapter I draw on the findings of a study in which I investigated the ward learning environment for student nurses and its relationship to the quality of nursing (Smith 1988). The nursing process emerged as an important component in understanding that relationship. At the time the study was undertaken (1983–85), nursing models were not clearly articulated as the conceptual basis on which nursing was taught and practised; the nursing process, with its associated framework of daily living activities (Henderson 1960, Roper 1976), served this function. A literature review showed that over the preceding decade the nursing process had been interpreted by nurse leaders and educationalists as both a device for organising nursing knowledge and a work method for improving standards of care. The nursing process appeared to be the forerunner of nursing models.

Little research had been undertaken to demonstrate how the nursing process operated in the everyday world of nurse practitioners and teachers. My study provided insights into the theory and practice of the nursing process in one school of nursing and its role in maintaining standards of patient care. Furthermore, the findings appeared to be relevant to an analysis of nursing models and their application to nurse education and practice.

This chapter is divided into two sections. The first section presents a summary of the nursing process literature. In the second I draw on research findings that address issues raised by that literature, in relation to the nursing process and the content and form of nurse training; the caring role of the nurse; and the maintenance of standards. Finally, I summarise the findings and raise questions about nursing models and their application to nurse education and practice.

The literature on the nursing process

I identified two influential papers that illustrated how nurse leaders promoted the nursing process; they were presented by Jean McFarlane, a leading nurse academic (1976, 1977). In the first she promoted 'a charter for caring' to the Royal College of Nursing, and in the second she presented a 'theory' for nursing to a conference for teachers of degree nursing programmes.

The first paper (McFarlane 1976) was a clear exposition of the central role of 'caring' in nursing. Reference was made to Henderson's activities of daily living and 'the unique function of the nurse' described in *Basic Principles of Nursing Care* (Henderson 1960), and to Orem's 'self-care' or daily living activities (1971). On the strength of these two nursing 'theorists' and the consensus view of the North America-based Nursing Development Conference Group (1973), McFarlane claimed that nursing was about 'helping, assisting, serving, caring' rather than acting as the stereotype doctor's assistant involved in cure.

McFarlane discussed the meaning of the words 'nursing' and 'caring' and maintained that they had similar roots: 'Caring signifies a feeling of concern, of interest, of oversight, with a view to protection. Nursing means ... to nourish and cherish.' She regretted an earlier job analysis of nursing that categorised the nurse's work as either 'basic' or 'technical' activity (Goddard 1953). 'Basic' work was subsequently relegated to unskilled activities undertaken by junior staff and relatives. The 'technical' work, seen as more 'prestigious' and 'complicated' and associated with medical treatment, was reserved for more experienced and senior staff. As a result, nurses would fail to appreciate the skill and complexity involved in undertaking 'basic' tasks such as bathing an aphasic patient with a stroke. McFarlane therefore believed that the 'caring role must be pre-eminent'. She did not refer in detail to the nursing process, but outlined the underlying theoretical models which she saw as appropriate to the central role of caring.

In the second paper (1977) she suggested: 'There is a call to systematise the practice of nursing and to record and analyse it (i.e. there is a need to document the nursing process.' She also outlined the observational and interviewing skills required to practise the nursing process. Repeated practice was recommended until the process became 'part of the nurse's approach and repertoire'. In that same year, the General Nursing Council for England and Wales included the nursing process in the general nursing training curriculum (1977). One of the first British textbooks on the subject was published in 1979 (Kratz) and described the nursing process as 'a problem-solving approach to nursing' based on four steps defined as assessment, planning, implementation and evaluation. The nursing process was also used by a Royal College of Nursing working group as the basis for setting standards of care (Royal College of Nursing 1980, 1981).

Armstrong (1983) argues that the nurse–patient relationship as constructed in standard nursing textbooks has changed dramatically since the introduction of the nursing process. The nurse's primary caring role was previously portrayed as concerned strictly with the patient's biological functioning. According to Armstrong, patients and, by inference, nurses were prevented from acknowledging and expressing their emotions. But from the mid-1970s, the textbooks changed their emphasis to psychology and communication skills, and 'subjectivity' entered the nurse–patient relationship. Armstrong refers to Kratz (1979) as one such example.

McFarlane remained firm in her view that nursing was a 'practice discipline' (1985); that its 'special domain is the daily living or self care activities contributing to health'; and that 'education for nursing needs to be soundly grounded in those skills and sciences that give insight into human functioning'. However, she doubted that the nurse education system, despite its stated commitment to the nursing process, was adequate to put into practice what she had outlined.

Changes in the way nursing is conceptualised have taken place in spite of McFarlane's pessimism, expressed both in 1977, when she noted the lack of nursing theories and concepts underpinning curriculum design, and again in 1985 as stated above. For example, nursing models were developed and refined from Henderson's activities of living by Roper (1976) and her colleagues Logan and Tierney (e.g. Roper, Logan & Tierney 1985). The original Roper model was derived from studies of clinical areas to which student nurses were allocated (Roper 1975). She observed students and patients and examined the nursing records to establish the learning context available on each ward. She discovered that patients' diagnostic labels sometimes differed from the designated specialty of the ward. It also appeared that any patient, irrespective of diagnosis, provided nurses with opportunities for unexpected teaching and learning. Overall, it was difficult to predict learning experience when allocation was based on the ward's medical specialty. Roper developed a patient profile instrument which could be used to define student learning and plan allocation related to patient dependency, using Henderson's activities of daily living rather than medical specialty. She concluded that student nurses' learning objectives and patterns of allocation should be planned using nursing rather than medical criteria.

Roper, Logan and Tierney (1985) offer an explanation for the development of nursing models to provide a more comprehensive theoretical framework for the practice of the nursing process: 'It was the wider application of the process in practice which confirmed for many nurses that the process is merely a *method* of carrying out nursing, but does not shed light on what comprises nursing'. Similarly, a series of articles in *Nursing Times* on nursing models and theories aimed to show how they can be used 'to create an informed basis for the use of the nursing process'. (The series has now been published in a book by Aggleton & Chalmers 1986.) The 'theories' referred to are described as 'conceptual models for practice' (Riehl & Roy 1980) and are in use in the curricula of the Diploma in Nursing and degree programmes.

Webb (1984) discovered that the nursing process had been superseded in many hospitals in the USA by nursing diagnoses and standardised, computerised care plans – and that nurse educationalists had grave misgivings about nursing 'theories', which are now referred to by the more modest term 'conceptual framework'. She also pointed out that these frameworks amounted to no more than 'a collection of unverified assumptions which reflect the personal philosophies or value-systems of their authors'.

Similarly, little substantive research has been undertaken in the UK to 'test' the viability of these 'frameworks' in the empirical reality. Miller (1985a) described the difficulties encountered by experienced nurses in relating nursing theories and models to their own practice, both verbally and in using them to write case studies for the Diploma in Nursing. She attributed these difficulties to the broad and abstract nature of the 'theories' and their complex language, which rendered them remote from reality. These nursing 'theories' appeared to offer limited insights into the nature of nursing as experienced in the everyday world of nurses and patients.

Keyzer (1985) evaluated the impact of the new curricula of the Diploma in Nursing and a nationally approved postbasic nursing course in the care of the elderly on the practice of the nursing process in four wards of four hospitals. His findings suggest that the implementation of the nursing process and the redefinition of the nurse's caring role is limited in the absence of supportive education programmes and a redistribution of power and control between patients and nurses, nurses and nurse managers, and nurses and doctors.

The nursing process appears to be more successful in its application to nursing practice as a work method, as shown by its use by nurses in a variety of settings (Miller 1985b). However, no systematic attempts are made by the authors she cites to evaluate its impact. How, then, did my research address the issues raised by the literature: the impact of the nursing process on the content and form of nurse training; the extent to which the caring role of the nurse has been redefined by the emphasis of the nursing process on subjectivity and interpersonal relationships; and its role in maintaining standards? I drew on findings based on a content analysis of training documents and timetables, interviews with nurse teachers and students and observation of classroom activities. The data were collected in a large teaching hospital during 1984 and 1985 (Smith 1987).

Impact of the nursing process on nurse training

I had found in the literature that the nursing process was portrayed both as a work method and as a way of organising nursing knowledge based on the activities of living, communication skills and a people-orientated approach to patient care. I therefore examined the content and form of nurse training in one school of nursing to assess the extent to which the nursing process as was applied in practice. The three-year course was divided into a foundation unit followed by 15 modules of approximately 10 weeks each. The modules offered students experience in medicine, surgery, paediatrics, obstetrics, geriatrics, gynaecology and psychiatry. Students were also allocated to the operating theatres and accident and emergency departments. During the first and third years there were two modules each of medicine and surgery (eight modules in all), suggesting that priority was given to students gaining experience in general/specialist medical and surgical nursing.

I studied a series of curriculum papers which presented the aims and/or objectives for the school-based content of training for each module. These aims and objectives reflected a commitment to meeting patients' physical, psychological and social needs: to planning, implementing and evaluating their care; and to acquiring management and teaching skills. However, the suggested content of the curriculum for meeting these aims and objectives was dominated by the natural sciences in the foundation unit and by the signs and symptoms, techniques and procedures associated with patients with medically defined conditions in subsequent modules. The nursing process as work method was mentioned by name twice in weeks two and three as suggested content for the foundation unit; it arose elsewhere in the curriculum by implication only. For example, its application to the care of patients in a medical or psychiatric setting was referred to as the need 'to plan, carry out and evaluate their total and integrated care'. The suggested content of the psychiatric module differed from that of general medicine in that it prioritised the 'psychological and social needs' of the patient.

During my interviews with students it emerged that once they had completed their first ward placement they criticised the natural science bias of the foundation unit: 'All cells and bits that don't connect with the patient' and 'A-level stuff ... which you never remember'. At this early stage the students readily described nursing in terms of activities of living such as bathing, lifting, feeding, toileting, talking and empathy with patients. They did not, however, automatically link these activities with the nursing process's underlying conceptual framework. Only two students described care and people as part of nursing knowledge, but they did not associate them with the conceptual base of the nursing process. Both were in the first six months of training. One student said about the concept of classroom teaching: 'Nothing is really said about care. They [the tutors] say you have to care but nobody actually says what caring is.' Another student said: 'School's got potential. Nursing isn't a dry boring subject ... we are talking about people.' After six months of training, students talked about knowing 'the basics by now' and 'needing to know more about different techniques and investigations'. Nursing theory was described as 'the solid facts, the diseases, the anatomy and physiology'.

The students' comments were indicative of a shift in emphasis during the first year away from assisting patients with living activities to the 'solid facts' of 'theory' and the techniques and procedures of practice. A third-year student illustrated this commitment to learning about 'facts' and a renewed interest in biological knowledge when she said: 'I am a third of the way through my third year and I don't know a massive amount. I did biology up to A-level so I do know how much I should know ... I want higher knowledge from the school ... somewhere the absolute facts are being missed out.' She was using A-level biology as a yardstick to measure the knowledge and 'absolute facts' she believed she needed to become a qualified nurse.

Although students did not identify the nursing process as part of the theoretical content of their training, they were able to conceptualise it as a work method based on ward experiences rather than on classroom abstractions. This finding is consonant with Miller's (1985b) findings. A first warder, when asked 'Did you learn about the nursing process in school?' said: 'We did a bit, but I don't think we realised how important it was. We didn't do a care plan until our last day in school, but if they [the tutors] had tied it up with the nursing process you would have realised that the two went together. But I didn't realise until then that that was the nursing process and that was what you did with it.' The same student was still having difficulty in describing the nursing process conceptually at the end of her third ward. After some thought she defined it as 'what do you do, really'. A third ward student assessed the nursing process as 'such a waffly subject... it all boils down to common sense in the end'.

Third year students described the nursing process in the following way: 'I would say it is patient allocation as opposed to work allocation . . . It's more thinking of the patient as a whole as opposed to one nurse being responsible for bedpans, etc.' Another much-quoted example was the use of the nursing process for obtaining written information about patients' technical care, as the following quotation illustrates: 'The nursing process is useful on surgical wards for telling you what dressings patients need and what to clean wounds with, etc., or on wards where the verbal reporting isn't very good.'

Thus the nursing process was seen as a work method rather than a way of organising nursing knowledge based on activities of living and communication skills. One reason for this appeared to be that tutors did not help the students to associate the nursing process with any underlying theoretical framework or nursing model. One tutor admitted she was uncertain about the nursing process approach to care: 'I do like the medical model and it can be nice and logical and it's scientific and you can do that in school beautifully. I don't think we can throw the medical model out completely because at the end of the day we have got people coming in [to hospital] with diseases.' She then described what she saw as a nursing model: 'I think the model becomes a bit pedantic. It's another checklist against which to tick off your knowledge or hang your concepts on. We have gone overboard thinking it's the person we must look at.' She concluded that: 'Nurse tutors are having difficulties using the nursing model. We haven't been sufficiently prepared.' The nursing process was about feelings and attitudes and more applicable to the ward. Another tutor who described herself as 'pro nursing process' described colleagues whose teaching was still 'very task orientated and based on the medical model'. Yet another thought that tutors were 'not good at equipping students with communication and interviewing skills which are fundamental to the nursing process'.

The tutors were more able than the students to conceptualise nursing in terms of activities of living and the nursing process, but they were still reluctant to replace the so-called medical model with a nursing one. They also felt subject to organisational constraints on the content of their teaching at both a national and a local level. For example, the curriculum was based on a syllabus external to the school (General Nursing Council for England and Wales 1977), mentioned by one tutor who confirmed that 'we teach the nursing process because it's in the syllabus'. Another tutor said: 'I'm a Jack of all trades and master of none. I teach 22 different subjects. Microbiology; they don't ask if I have a microbiology degree. They ask you to teach pharmacology. What do I know about pharmaceuticals? – All sorts of things.' This tutor was describing not only the subject areas that the content of the plan of training covered (i.e. medically oriented) but also the dilemma of the nurse teacher as generalist rather than specialist, who lacked control over the topics she taught and consequently did not teach nursing.

Redefining the nurse's caring role

To what extent had the introduction of the nursing process to nurse training redefined the caring role of the nurse as described by Armstrong (1983)? I observed a number of classes and undertook a content analysis of selected modules.

The tutors' reluctance to dispense with the medical model, and their feelings of constraint, were reflected in the content of their teaching. Analysis of the foundation unit and medical module timetables for a group of first and third year students confirmed that preference was given to sessions associated with biological science, medical specialities and technical procedures. Affective/psychosocial nursing (communication skills, activities of daily living) and the nursing process accounted for only 14% of sessions.

Following Armstrong's suggestion that 'subjectivity' had entered the nurse–patient relationship, I assumed that the formal training of students to care emotionally for patients was most likely to occur during those sessions categorised as affective/psychosocial nursing. Non-participant observation of a classroom session on death and dying yielded some insights. It was led by a tutor (T) who was completing a counselling course and was interested in how students (S) managed their emotions. Talking about working on the oncology wards, one student said:

S: You get to lay out so many people, you know how to do it. It's gruelling, horrible, but I'm not so afraid of death now.

T: Who helped?

S: One of the staff nurses. You become so blasé on a ward like that.

S: Nurses on the oncology wards, it's ruining their career, the involvement with patients becomes too much. They're now hard.

S: You feel cheated when a patient you've looked after dies while you're off duty.

S: The trained staff just don't want to know.

T: They need to develop counselling skills and build up support.

This account draws attention to strategies for dealing with death and dying by which nurses become 'blasé' and 'hard'. Students suggested that nurses needed to maintain empathy with patients, describing 'over-involvement' and subsequent 'hardness' as ruining staff nurses' careers. It appeared that the lack of training in techniques for managing emotions was seen to result in a withdrawal of emotional care. As first-year students, nurses still wanted involvement with patients and felt cheated if those with whom they were involved died when they were not on duty. The trained staff 'not wanting to know' again suggested withdrawal of emotional care by failing to acknowledge the students' feelings about the deaths.

Emotional issues were discussed by the tutor who led the session, but she did not offer the students specific training in techniques to manage their feelings. She acknowledged that trained staff on the oncology ward needed to develop counselling skills to offer support to others, but she did not develop the discussion.

The psychiatric module towards the end of the second year went some way towards training students to care for patients emotionally. The module was identified by general tutors and students as having an important role in developing communication skills and psychological understanding. A student confirmed this when she said about her psychiatric experience: 'It taught me a lot, I think. It teaches you a lot about the importance of talking to your patients and that sort of psychological side of their care ... I think you are much more aware of it.' Other than the psychiatric module, the limited number of sessions categorised as 'psychosocial nursing' suggests that students received little formal training in emotional care. Rather, the presence of affective/psychosocial sessions put students under added pressure to give emotional care to patients, without the necessary skills. The psychiatric module attempted to rectify this, but since it lasted only nine weeks its long-term effects were probably of limited value (Collister 1983).

The majority of students, however, thought that they learned communication skills informally, through role modelling and experience, and not in the classroom. A student who had just taken her state final examination said that she learned by watching other people and identifying 'a good model'. She continued: 'You think "I'll remember that", or "that's not the way I'd do it". Then again it's almost inspirational or off-the-cuff. You think, "I've never met this before; I've got to act". Or you go off duty and think how you handle something and sift through it.'

Third warders commented: 'You can't be taught to react ... I think if you want to talk about things [like death], you usually talk about it to your friends when you come off duty.'

'Sometimes you do need support with very confused patients. You need someone [at night] to be able to turn to and say "what do I do?".'

'It comes with practice anyway. The more you come in contact with, say, violent patients, you learn how to cope with that yourself because that's how the third years have learned ... just through experience.'

Many of the students considered that they were already able to communicate with others because of the sort of people they themselves were and what had motivated them to come into nursing. A first year student said: 'You have to be able, even as a first warder, to have the character to be able to talk to strangers, and very quickly. If you haven't got that I don't think you can nurse well.'

About the nursing process and communication skills, another first year student said: 'I think that if you're basically a sort of caring person, which presumably you are if you come into nursing, then I think you've your own sort of procedure. I don't think you should try and make everyone the "standard" nurse.'

Both these comments reflected the predominant ideology of nursing as care work.

Role of the nursing process in maintaining standards

Further analysis of the plan of training revealed that students underwent 'a planned series of structured and informal assessments based on detailed objectives'. These assessments were described as 'a means by which encouragement is given to learners to *reach and maintain high standards of nursing care throughout training'* (my italics).

The students were given clinical learning objectives related to wards and specialities. These objectives reflected those stated in the curriculum and were concerned with acquiring competence in techniques and procedures associated with the care of patients suffering from specific diseases. Relatively few objectives were identified concerning affective or psychosocial care.

The principal means of testing skills and related knowledge were said to be practical assessment and ward reports. Attitudes were also said to be tested by ward reports and professional appraisal. Nurse teachers were designated as assessors of written work and professionalism, and trained staff as assessors of nursing skills. There was a formal assessment of nursing skills in nine out of 15 modules, based on medical specialities, which included the assessment of specific procedures such as aseptic technique. In module 12, the criteria for the assessment of nursing skills were stated as 'the observation of planning and organisation of care given by the student and colleagues; the *quality of care* given by students and colleagues; and the written and verbal reports related to plan of care when carried out' (my italics).

The format of the assessment of nursing skills was based on the nursing process framework of assessment, planning, implementation of care plan, and evaluation. However, the nursing process was not referred to by name. Criteria on which the nurse was assessed included 'personal appearance' as well as communication with patients and an awareness of cultural, spiritual, physical and psychological needs. She was also expected to be able to prioritise care, ensure safety at all times, record and report care given, evaluate care in terms of its effects on patients, use teaching opportunities and evaluate her own performance. The content of the assessment was based on the student's level of training. Thus, a first warder would be assessed on the care of one patient only, whereas a third-year was judged on her ability to manage both patients and colleagues. Additionally, the ward report at the end of every allocation judged students on similar criteria, and on women's traditional attributes as described by Ungerson (1983). These attributes included appearance, punctuality, observation, forethought, identification of priorities and a high level of social skills.

Thus methods of assessment (especially ward reports), couched in the language of the nursing process, set the tone for a more subjective approach to patient care and a means by which pressure was put on students to maintain standards. One student said about the assessments: 'In this hospital there is a very definite attempt to make you change your character ... well ... mould you into a "City" type.' The student went on to describe one ward sister as the 'City type': She's everybody's ideal really. She's so sophisticated, she always looks so calm, attractive and manages to get all the work done [and] she's very kind and considerate and yet she looks almost like a model ... I think the standards and ideals are very high here: what they want you to be.' I asked, 'Who are *they*?' She replied, 'School and the staff nurses, I suppose. I don't know who formulates the ward reports ... a list of all the qualities you should have. You get marks on them. It's whoever draws up that who is moulding you.'

Another student expressed similar views: 'The reports give you a picture of what *they* [the trained staff] think you are like, not like I think I am.'

Thus it appeared that at this school the language of the nursing process had been used to help formulate the students' practical assessments and make them conform to certain behaviour patterns. Feelings and emotions in nurse–patient relations had been made visible and the tone had been set for maintaining high standards of nursing.

Medical concepts or nursing concepts?

My findings confirm that medical rather than nursing concepts continued to dominate the content of nurse training in this school of nursing. The theoretical and practical content of the three-year programme were organised around medical rather than nursing specialities as described by Roper (1975). Even though the nursing process was represented in the language of the plan of training, it had not been adopted by either students or tutors as a viable 'theoretical' alternative to the 'medical model'.

The tutors expressed verbal commitment to the nursing process as a device for teaching and learning nursing. However, they had no theoretical framework on which to base their teaching. For example, there was no evidence to suggest that they were explicitly using nursing models and 'theories' as a means of conceptualising nursing (Aggleton & Chalmers 1986). In practice the tutors fell back on, and their teaching programmes were overshadowed by, subjects that promoted the acquisition of medical knowledge and technical skills. Students described the nursing process as a work method rather than in terms suggesting an underlying conceptual framework of living activities and communication skills.

The nursing process, however, had introduced feelings and emotions into the patient–nurse relationship as suggested by Armstrong (1983), and had increased the visibility of emotional care as a component of nursing. The terminology used to underpin the plan of training and regular assessments encouraged students to 'maintain high standards of nursing', and could be interpreted as the means by which they were put under pressure to meet patients' emotional and other needs. However, it appeared that nurses were inadequately trained or supported in techniques essential to managing the complexity of emotional care.

To conclude, the nursing process as work method and nursing models as 'theory' have not yet offered a viable alternative to the organisation of nurse training based on medical facts, although they have raised the profile of nursing as care work. One reason appears to be that the versions of nursing they offer fail to address the emotional and structural complexities of the nursing labour process and the training and supervision of students in school and ward. The viability of nursing models will therefore remain in question until these complexities are considered in the development of a knowledge base that reflects the everyday reality of nursing work and learning.

Acknowledgements

I would like to express my gratitude to the nurses and patients who made this research possible, and to Bloomsbury Health Authority who supported it.

References

Aggleton P & Chalmers H (1986) *Nursing Models and the Nursing Process.* London: Macmillan.

Armstrong D (1983) The fabrication of nurse–patient relationships. *Social Science and Medicine*, **17**(8), 457–460.

Collister B (1983) The value of psychiatric experience in general nurse training. *Nursing Times*, Occasional Paper, **79**(29), 66–69.

General Nursing Council for England and Wales (1977) *Training Syllabus Register of Nurses: General Nursing.* London: GNC.

Goddard H (1953) *The Work of Nurses in Hospital Wards: Report of a Job Analysis.* London: Nuffield Provincial Hospitals Trust.

Henderson V (1960) *Basic Principles of Nursing Care.* Geneva: International Council of Nurses.

Keyzer D (1985) *Learning Contracts, the Trained Nurse and the Implementation of the Nursing Process: Comparative Case Studies in the Management of Knowledge and Change in Nursing Practice.* PhD thesis, University of London.

Kratz C, ed. (1979) *The Nursing Process.* London: Baillière Tindall.

McFarlane J (1976) A charter for caring. *Journal of Advanced Nursing*, **1,** 187–196.

McFarlane J (1977) Developing a theory of nursing: the relation of theory to practice, education and research. *Journal of Advanced Nursing,* **2**(3), 261–270.

McFarlane J (1985) Contemporary challenges in education for the caring professions: education for nursing, midwifery and health visiting. *British Medical Journal,* **291,** 263–271.

Miller A (1985a) The relationship between nursing theory and nursing practice. *Journal of Advanced Nursing,* **10**(5), 417–424.

Miller A (1985b) Does the process help the patient? *Nursing Times,* **81**(26), 24–27.

Nursing Development Conference Group (1973) *Concept Formalisation in Nursing.* Boston: Little, Brown.

Orem D (1971) *Nursing: Concepts of Practice.* New York: McGraw-Hill.

Riehl J & Roy C, eds (1980) *Conceptual Models for Nursing Practice.* Norwalk, CT: Appleton Century Crofts.

Roper N (1975) *Clinical Experience in Nurse Education: A Survey of the Available Nursing Experience for General Student Nurses in a School of Nursing in Scotland.* MPhil thesis, University of Edinburgh.

Roper N (1976) A model for nursing and nursology. *Journal of Advanced Nursing,* **1**(3), 219–227.

Roper N, Logan W & Tierney A (1985) The Roper/Logan/Tierney model. *Senior Nurse,* **3**(2), 20–26.

Royal College of Nursing (1980) *Standards of Nursing Care.* London: RCN.

Royal College of Nursing (1981) *Towards Standards.* London: RCN.

Smith P (1987) The relationship between quality of nursing care and the ward as a learning environment: developing a methodology. *Journal of Advanced Nursing*, **12,** 413–420.

Smith P (1988) *Quality of Nursing and the Ward as a Learning Environment for Student Nurses: A Multimethod Approach.* PhD thesis, University of London.

Ungerson C (1983) Women and caring: skills, tasks and taboos. In Gamarnikov E, Morgan D, Purvis J & Taylorson D, eds. *The Public and the Private.* London: Heinemann.

Webb C (1984) On the eighth day God created the nursing process and nobody rested. *Senior Nurse,* **1**(33), 22–25.

Models for Nursing 2
Edited by B Kershaw and J Salvage
© 1990 Scutari Press

13
Towards 2000

BETTY KERSHAW

The development of models of nursing spread from the USA to the UK in the early 1980s, yet their use in nursing practice is still patchy in the UK. Many clinical nurses consider them a ploy introduced by nurse theoreticians to add to the mystification of a simple activity: the practice of nursing (see Chapman's evidence for these arguments in Chapter 2 of this book). There are many reasons behind such a criticism. As Wright (1986) reports, the use of a model has often been imposed with little or no discussion with practitioners. The model selected may not always be suitable for all patients, yet there may be no variation to take account of individual need. The use of the model may be 'routinised' in much the same way as the nursing process. Such practices negate the whole purpose of using a model of nursing.

Elements of a model for nursing practice

In view of these problems it is important to reiterate the elements of a model for nursing practice and the purpose of using it. Roy (1984) lists the essential elements as:

- a description of the person receiving care;
- a statement of the goal of nursing;
- a definition of health;
- a specified meaning of environment;
- a delineation of nursing activities.

127

A description of the person receiving care

To describe her patient fully the nurse needs to assess him: to carry out the first stage of nursing process. Nurses may find assessment difficult and must take care to note what they observe or find out rather than make assumptions based on medical diagnosis, age, social class, gender and so on. The model chosen frequently directs the way the assessment is carried out. For example, a nurse using Orem's model will be required to analyse her patient's self-care deficits. These may be developmental. For example, a young child cannot feed himself and needs someone to assist with this activity. Or the deficit may be caused by ill-health: an adult suffering from burns to the hands may also have difficulty in feeding himself. He has a self-care deficit and needs help with eating until he can use his hands again. A nurse using an adaptation model of nursing (such as Roy 1984) will identify maladaptive health perspectives and the reasons why these have arisen. Thus she would identify tiredness, breathlessness and pallor in a patient whose diet was poor in nutrients, especially iron.

Whichever model she uses, the nurse needs to ensure that problems are identified from the patient's perspective. There are occasions when a nurse may perceive that a problem or a need is present, but the patient does not agree. A frequently quoted example is the patient who 'lives rough'; to the nurse he has several 'self-care deficits' and is exhibiting 'maladaptation'. However, many other patients value their independence from what they see as interference in meeting their needs.

Statement of the goal of nursing

The way in which the model is formulated affects the way in which the goals for nursing care are specified. For example, the goals may be described in terms of achieving a level of self-care or adaptation. These terms can themselves create problems. Is it possible that the concept of self-care may be used as an excuse to reduce the level of nursing care? Do patients subject to a self-care approach feel neglected by nurses? What about the public expectations that nurses give care? And does accepting adaptation as a goal imply to patients and nurses that improvement is no longer possible? A nurse using a model to plan and give care must ensure that her patients and their families and friends understand the philosophy. The model she chooses should be appropriate for that patient, and the goals of the institution (for example, adherence to a self-care model) should not replace those most appropriate for the patient. She must also take care not to act in a manner which assumes that the professional view is best.

Definition of health

One of the criticisms of models of nursing is that they give no definitive statement of health. This is not entirely fair, as the ability to function in any given setting such as that defined by the model may imply a social definition of health. Most people would define health as a state of complete physical, social and psychological well-being. However, not everyone who considers himself healthy fits this definition; the farmer with insulin-dependent diabetes, or the school teacher who works from a wheelchair and lives with her family in a specially adapted bungalow, would both see themselves as healthy. A model should make its definition overt, not covert, and include provision for health education and health promotion. Neuman (1982) sees health as 'the stability of the system', and Rogers (1970) defines it as a 'feeling of wholeness'; both are vague about health outcomes, but their definitions are at least visible in their work. Perhaps the best definitions of health are given by Rogers, who explores several perspectives.

Specified meaning of environment

Probably no word has been so overworked in recent years as 'environment'. Normally it is used in a very broad context and relates to natural phenomena. However, all of us are situated in a more intimate environment within this larger setting – our home, place of work, or hospital. The setting in which a patient is living alters his needs, his adaptation levels and self-care deficits, and may alter the goals that are set. The model may need to be chosen with a particular setting in mind; some models are seen to be more appropriate for use in one environment than another.

Delineation of nursing activities

It is not always appreciated that models are not restricted to nurses. Many aspects of models are relevant to care given by other members of the team, such as physiotherapists. Wright (1986) describes the use of his nursing model and the associated documentation and care-giving by all members of the multi-disciplinary team, but it must always be the nurse using the nursing model who indicates how care should be given to achieve the goals of nursing practice.

Models define each of these essential elements individually. They also demonstrate how they interact. A model is therefore able to portray a whole set of related concepts or activities at one time. This allows the person using it to visualise the effect of actions not yet carried out, and the way variation in practice will alter the outcome of nursing activities. As McFarlane (1986) argued, models may:

● serve as a tool that links theory and practice;
● clarify thinking about the elements of a practice situation and their relationship to each other;
● help practitioners of nursing communicate with each other more meaningfully;
● serve as a guide to practice, education and research.

The future: poised for change

The future of nursing practice and education is poised for change. As we move towards the next century we will see many more people receiving care in their own homes from relatives, friends and volunteers. Government policies, economic factors, patients' wishes and a reduction in trained nurses will all hasten these changes, which will mean a change in the nurse's role and function – away from direct giver of care and towards care planner and facilitator. The educational changes set out in Project 2000, the UK Central Council for Nursing, Midwifery and Health Visiting's strategy for nursing education, aim to prepare the nurse for this new role (UKCC 1986). The 'new nurse' will be 'a knowledge-able doer' able to give skilled nursing care built on a sound theoretical know-ledge base. This improved knowledge base must include an understanding of nursing theories and models and how to apply them to clinical practice. Wright (1985) has described the role of the English National Board for Nursing, Midwifery and Health Visiting in introducing models into the curriculum. Its requirement that colleges should introduce model-based curricula, without accompanying changes in the clinical areas used for placements, has increased the confusion that many students experience when trying to relate nursing theory to nursing practice. Like many other experienced nurses, Wright recognises that it is inadequate simply to teach about models; it is their application to practice that will cause them to be valued and developed.

Nurse teachers must therefore not only improve their own knowledge of nursing models, but must also become skilled in assisting clinical nurses to apply them to practice. This need for development of nurse teachers is being recog-nised by committees of the national boards and professional organisations which are looking at the content of courses to update teachers for Project 2000. The UKCC, in proposing rules for Project 2000 courses (1988a), moves on from the ENB guidance by stating that, in order to provide a knowledge base, the follow-ing subjects should be explored during the 18-month common foundation programme: 'Theory and Practice of Nursing: values; concepts; ideologies; models; information systems; research methodology and application.' It would like teachers to ensure that students are able to 'demonstrate application of care knowledge and skills during supervised and specified experience in practice settings.' By the time the student enters her second 18 months of training, she should be developing previous CFP learning and also exploring 'theoretical frameworks' and models of care within the settings appropriate to the branch being studied. It is therefore essential that nurse teachers assist the development of model-based practice.

Clinical staff, too, must be given the opportunity to acquire similar skills in con-tinuing education courses. A second paper from the UKCC (1988b) discusses the content of programmes for nurses returning to work after a break. Suggestions for course outcomes include 'the ability to design, execute and evaluate plans of patient/client care based on appropriate models'. There is surely an obligation on teachers and managers to ensure that this ability is also developed by nurses who have remained in practice.

Many nurses who are using models in practice have developed these skills as part of degree and diploma work. It is interesting to note the influence of advanced nursing courses in the use of models, since the plans for nursing educa-tion envisage a much closer affiliation between higher education institutions and schools of nursing. This should facilitate the application of theory to practice, since nurses who understand the rationale underlying nursing action are much more likely to implement new ideas.

The introduction of nursing models into Project 2000 curricula will be a matter for individual schools of nursing, taking into consideration the philosophies of their health authorities and affiliated institutions. It may prove easier to follow what is already established practice in many schools, introducing the student in the early stages (the common foundation programme?) to a 'simplistic' model, and moving on to explore clinical application in the branch programmes. At postbasic and degree level, students can be encouraged to criticise the work of newer theorists, expand this to meet the needs of their own patients, and develop their own philosophical framework for practice. So much is possible!

The registered nurse will be supported by the care assistant or support worker. It is not yet clear what preparation will be offered for the role, but training is clearly needed to enable her to assist the nurse with care-giving. To ensure that the patient does not suffer from fragmentation of care, all involved must communicate effectively with one another, share common goals (agreed with the patient), and work to achieve them in a coordinated way. A model of nursing could assist in all these requirements.

Working together in practice

How can this work in practice? Consider the case of Mr Brown, aged 65, who had a mid-thigh amputation for circulatory failure. His primary nurse discussed his care and postoperative progress with him; they agreed that the desired outcome of treatment was that he should return to normal life as soon as possible. In view of this aim, Orem's model of self-care was selected as the most appropriate framework for planning his care. This model recognises that there is a continuum of self-care ability. Immediately postoperatively the nurse had to meet most of the patient's demands. However, once he became conscious he became involved in his own self-care, with the nurse acting for him only where he was unable to function – thus making good any self-care deficit.

Mobility was obviously a problem in the early days, but with help from the nurse and teaching from the physiotherapist Mr Brown was able to sit out of bed. Due to hospital policy and the wishes of the patient and his wife, he was discharged home five days after the operation. The nurse who visited him at home and the physiotherapist in the department he visited daily needed to understand the level of mobility he had reached on discharge and the goals set. The model assisted in this, as the plan of care and the goals originally drawn up by the primary nurse and the patient could be used by the visiting nurse and the physiotherapist. Updating was carried out as early goals of self-care were reached; as Mr Brown progressed to a well-fitting artificial limb, it was possible to see how he had moved along the continuum from total self-care deficit to independence and ability to meet his own needs.

One model is not suitable for all patients. Mrs Smith, aged 34, was diagnosed as having a rapidly progressive muscular dystrophy. When first seen as an outpatient she was able to walk, though rather unsteadily, but her condition deteriorated and the community nurse was called in. On her first visit the nurse assessed her current abilities and needs, and in discussion with Mrs Smith worked out a plan that would enable her to remain at home and independent as long as possible. Both nurse and patient realised that this would require changes in care in order to meet her changing abilities; they decided to use Roy's adaptation model as a framework for action.

Helping the patient to function to the best of her ability required changes in the expectations of the family members, who all contributed to make up for her declining competence. The house was adapted to allow free movement of a wheelchair; aids were supplied to enable her to feed herself; relatives and friends were encouraged to take her out in the car, and when such outings became too difficult, to visit and include her in their plans and gossip. Her two children were encouraged to make the room in which she spent most of the day the centre of family activities, and were encouraged to bring in friends just as they would have done with a mother who was fit. Although the process was one of deterioration, the model focused attention on the way things could be achieved rather than on the fact that they were difficult. The visiting nurse had a large role to play in educating the family in how they too needed to adapt, and what they could do to help care for Mrs Smith.

As can be seen from these examples, no one model is appropriate for every situation. Sometimes the model may need to be changed to take account of changing needs, or an entirely new model formulated. With the changes that are likely to occur as a result of developments in medical science, the pressures of economic policy, the changing demands of the population, the shortage of young people and the corresponding increase in the number of the elderly, there will have to be changes in the patterns of nursing practice. A model may be used to demonstrate the interrelationships of these and other factors, and therefore to assist in understanding the situation, communicating the facts to others and ensuring that all share common goals.

Project 2000 recommends a common foundation programme of 18 months which will provide a firm theoretical base in biological and behavioural sciences as well as interpersonal skills, communication and nursing care. Experience will be provided in a wide range of clinical areas in institutional and community settings. A model of nursing linked with an appropriate curriculum model will help the student make sense of these experiences. As Wright (1986) says: 'In such a world of change how can nurses change themselves and bring order to what they do? It is in the construction of models that a large part of the answer lies, in helping to structure thinking and actions, to determine what a nurse needs to know in order to nurse, and to decide upon the best ways of putting nursing knowledge into practice.'

References

McFarlane J (1986) The value of models for care. In Kershaw B & Salvage J, eds. *Models for Nursing.* Chichester: John Wiley.

Neuman B (1982) *The Neuman Systems Model: Application to Nursing Education and Practice.* Norwalk, CT: Appleton Century Crofts.

Orem D (1980) *Nursing: Concepts of Practice.* 2nd edn. New York: McGraw-Hill.

Rogers M (1970) *An Introduction to the Theoretical Basis of Nursing.* Philadelphia: Davis.

Roy C (1984) *Introduction to Nursing: An Adaptation Model.* 2nd edn. Englewood Cliffs, NJ: Prentice Hall.

UKCC (1986) *Project 2000: a New Preparation for Practice.* London: UKCC.

UKCC (1988a) *Proposed Rules for the Standard, Kind and Content of Future Pre-registration Nursing Education.* Consultation paper. London: UKCC.

UKCC (1988b) *Proposals for a Statutory Requirement for Nurses and Health Visitors to Undertake Re-Entry programmes Prior to their Return to Practice.* Consultation paper. London: UKCC.

Wright S (1985) Strategy for change. *Senior Nurse*, **3**(34), 24–25.

Wright S (1986) *Building and Using a Model for Nursing.* London: Edward Arnold.

Selected Bibliography

Aggleton P & Chalmers H (1986) *Nursing Models and the Nursing Process.* London: Macmillan.

Aggleton P & Chalmers H (1987) Models of nursing, nursing practice and nurse education. *Journal of Advanced Nursing,* **12**(5), 573–581.

Barber P, ed. (1987) *Mental Handicap: Facilitating Holistic Care.* Sevenoaks. Hodder & Stoughton.

Barker J (1984) A plan for Arthur and Mary. *Nursing Times,* **80,** Community Outlook, 403–408.

Benner P (1984) *From Novice to Expert – Excellence and Power in Clinical Nursing Practice.* Menlo Park, CA: Addison Wesley.

Campbell C (1984) Orem's story. *Nursing Mirror,* **15**(13), 28–30.

Casey A (1988) A partnership for child and family. *Senior Nurse,* **8**(4), 8–9.

Chance K (1982) Nursing models: a requisite for professional accountability. *Advances in Nursing Science,* January, 57–65.

Chapman P (1984) Specifics and generalities: a critical examination of two nursing models. *Nurse Education Today,* **4**(6), 141–144.

Cheetham T (1988) Model care in the surgical ward. *Senior Nurse,* **8**(4), 10–12.

Chenitz C & Swanson J (1985) *From Practice to Grounded Theory.* New York: Addison Wesley.

Clark J (1982) Development of models and theories on the concept of nursing. *Journal of Advanced Nursing,* **7**(2), 129–134.

Cronenwett L (1983) Helping and nursing models. *Nursing Research,* **32**(6), 342–346.

Crow R (1982) Frontiers of nursing in the 21st century: development of models and theories on the concept of nursing. *Journal of Advanced Nursing,* **7**(2), 111–116.

Dyer J (1980) A model of care. *Nursing Mirror,* 24 April, 28–30.

Dylak P (1986) The state of the art. *Nursing Times,* **82**(42), 72.

Fawcett J (1980). A framework for analysis and evaluation of conceptual models of nursing. *Nurse Educator,* **5**(6), 553–558.

Fawcett J (1984) *Analysis and Evaluation of Conceptual Models of Nursing.* Philadelphia: Davis.

Foster D (1987) The development of care plans for the critically ill patient. *Nursing,* 3(15), 571–573.

George J (1985) *Nursing Theories: the Base for Professional Practice.* Englewood Cliffs, NJ: Prentice Hall.

Glasper E (1986) Scaling down a model. *Nursing Times,* **82**(43), 57–58.

Glasper E, Stonehouse J & Martin L (1987). Core care plans. *Nursing Times,* **83**(10), 55–57.

Green C (1985) An overview of the value of nursing models in relation to education. *Nurse Education Today,* **5**(6), 267–271.

Gruending D (1985) Nursing theory: a vehicle for professionalisation? *Journal of Advanced Nursing,* **10**(6), 553–558.

Hardy L (1982) Nursing models and research – a restricting view? *Journal of Advanced Nursing,* **7**(5), 447–451.

Hardy L (1986) Identifying the place of theoretical frameworks in an evolving discipline. *Journal of Advanced Nursing,* **11**(1), 103–107.

Hardy M (1978) Perspectives on nursing theory. *Advances in Nursing Science,* **1**, 37–48.

Henderson V (1960) *Basic Principles of Nursing Care.* Geneva: International Council of Nurses.

Henderson V (1966) *The Nature of Nursing.* London: Collier Macmillan.

Johnson D (1974) Development of theory: a requisite for nursing as a primary health profession. *Nursing Research,* **23**(5), 372–377.

Johnson M (1985) Model of perfection. *Nursing Times,* **82**(6), 42–44.

Kagan C M, ed. (1985) *Interpersonal Skills in Nursing: Research and Applications.* Beckenham: Croom Helm.

Kapelli S (1986) Nurses' management of patients' self care. *Nursing Times,* **82**(11), 40–43.

Katz F (1969) Nurses. In Etzioni A, ed., *The Semi-Professions and their Organisations.* USA: Free Press.

Kershaw B & Salvage J, eds (1986) *Models for Nursing.* Chichester: John Wiley.

Keyzer D (1985) *Learning Contracts, the Trained Nurse and the Implementation of the Nursing Process: Comparative Case Studies in the Management of Knowledge and Change in Nursing Practice.* Unpublished PhD thesis, University of London.

King I (1981) *A Theory of Nursing.* Chichester: John Wiley.

Kratz C, ed. (1979) *The Nursing Process.* London: Baillière Tindall.

Lauer P, Murphy S & Powers M (1982) Learning needs of cancer patients: a comparison of nurse and patient perceptions. *Nursing Research,* **31**(1), 11–16.

Lister P (1987) The misunderstood model. *Nursing Times,* **83**(41), 40–42.

Luker K (1988) Do models work? *Nursing Times,* **84**(5), 24–29.

Martin L & Glasper E (1986) Core plans – nursing models and the nursing process in action. *Nursing Practice,* **1**(4), 268–273.

Maslow A (1943) A theory of human motivation. *Psychological Review,* **50**, 370–396.

McFarlane J (1977) Developing a theory of nursing: the relation of theory to practice, education and research. *Journal of Advanced Nursing.* **2**(3), 261–270.

Meleis A (1985) *Theoretical Nursing,* London: Lippincott.

Midgley C (1988) *The Use of Models for Nursing within Midwifery Training Hospitals in England.* Unpublished paper, Huddersfield Polytechnic.

Miller A (1985) Does the process help the patient? *Nursing Times,* **81**(26), 24–27.

Miller A (1985) Theories in nursing. *Nursing Times,* **8**(10), 14.

Miller A (1985) The relationship between nursing theory and nursing practice. *Journal of Advanced Nursing,* **10**(5), 417–424.

Minshull J, Ross K & Turner J (1986) The human needs model of nursing. *Journal of Advanced Nursing,* **11**(6), 643–649.

Neuman B (1982) *The Neuman Systems Model: Application to Nursing Education and Practice*. Norwalk, CT: Appleton Century Crofts.

Newman M (1979) *Theory Development in Nursing*. Philadelphia: Davis.

Nursing Development Conference Group (1973) *Concept Formalisation in Nursing*. Boston: Little, Brown.

Orem D (1985) *Nursing: Concepts of Practice*. New York: McGraw-Hill.

Orlando I (1987) Nursing in the 21st century – alternative paths. *Journal of Advanced Nursing,* **12**(5), 405–412.

Pearson A (1985) Nurses as change agents, and the strategy for change. *Nursing Practice,* **1**(2), 80–84.

Pearson A & Vaughan B (1986) *Nursing Models for Practice*. London: Heinemann.

Peplau H (1952) *Interpersonal Relations in Nursing*. New York: Pitman.

Rambo B (1984) *Adaptation Nursing*. New York: Saunders.

Reilly D (1975) Why a conceptual framework? *Nursing Outlook,* **23**(9), 565–599.

Riehl J and Roy C, eds (1980) *Conceptual Models for Nursing Practice*. Norwalk, CT: Appleton Century Crofts.

Rogers M (1970) *An Introduction to the Theoretical Basis of Nursing,* Philadelphia: Davis.

Roper N (1976) A model for nursing and nursology. *Journal of Advanced Nursing* **1**(3), 219–227.

Roper N, Logan W & Tierney A (1983) *Using a Model for Nursing*. Edinburgh: Churchill Livingstone.

Roper N, Logan W & Tierney A (1985a) *The Elements of Nursing*. Edinburgh: Churchill Livingstone.

Roper N, Logan W and Tierney A (1985b) The Roper/Logan/Tierney model. *Senior Nurse,* **3**(2), 20–26.

Roy C (1984) *Introduction to Nursing: an Adaptation Model,* 2nd edn. Englewood Cliffs, NJ: Prentice Hall.

Royal College of Nursing (1980) *Standards of Nursing Care*. London: RCN.

Royal College of Nursing (1981) *Towards Standards*. London: RCN.

Silva M & Rothbart D (1984) An analysis of changing trends in philosophies of science on nursing theory development and testing. *Advances in Nursing Science,* **6**(2), 1–13.

Stevens B (1984) *Nursing Theory: Analysis, Application, Evaluation*. Boston: Little, Brown.

Torres G (1985) The place of concepts and theories within nursing. In George J, ed., *Nursing Theories*. Englewood Cliffs, NJ: Prentice Hall.

Travelbee J (1971) *Interpersonal Aspects of Nursing*. Philadelphia: Davis.

United Kingdom Central Council for Nursing, Midwifery and Health Visiting (1986) *Project 2000: a New Preparation for Practice*. London: UKCC.

Walsh M (1985) *Accident and Emergency Nursing: a New Approach*. London: Heinemann.

Weatherstone L (1979) Theory of nursing: creating effective care. *Journal of Advanced Nursing,* **4,** 365–375.

Webb C (1984) On the eighth day God created the nursing process and nobody rested. *Senior Nurse,* **1**(32), 22–25.

Wilding C, Wells M & Wilson I (1988) A model for family care. *Nursing Times,* **84**(15), 38, 40–41.

Wright S (1985) Change in nursing: the application of change theory to practice. *Nursing Practice.* **1**(2), 85–91.

Wright S (1985) Strategy for change. *Senior Nurse,* **3**(34), 24–25.

Wright S (1986) *Building and Using a Model of Nursing.* London: Edward Arnold.

Young W B (1987) *Introduction to Nursing Concepts.* California: Appleton & Large.

Yura H and Walsh M (1988) *The Nursing Process.* Norwalk, CT: Appleton Century Crofts.

Index

General Nursing Council for England
and Wales (GNC) 57–8, 116, 120
Goals 11, 48, 53, 79, 84, 96, 109
common 19, 71, 132
goal-directed care 50
inappropriate 41
of nursing 86, 127–9
patient 42–3
setting of 6, 31, 33, 42–3, 131
Gunzburg's inventory 80

Health 13–14, 69, 80–4, 86, 103, 127
concept of 24
definition of 81, 128–9
department of 58
and midwifery practice 60, 62
problem 70
promotion of 78
Health authority 40, 57, 75, 78, 90,
131
Health care 29–31, 47, 71, 103
consumers 11
organisation 69
professionals 47, 69–70
service 105
workers 104, 110, 112
Health education 26, 70, 91, 129
Health service ombudsman 26
Health visitor 26, 72
Henderson's conceptual framework
90–6, 100
needs identified 94
Henderson's concept of nursing 84, 91
Hierarchical structure 6, 105, 109, 111
and imposition of change 23–5, 40,
60
Holistic approach 49–50, 77–8, 80–1,
103, 129
and Henderson's model 93
Hospices 73–5
Hospitals 9, 14, 58, 72
district general 89
Human needs approach 60–2, 80, 93

Independence 48, 51, 78–80, 86, 131
and behavioural equilibrium 81
continua 84
encouragement of 84, 93
Individualised care 43–4, 50, 60, 89,
95
Informal carers 22

Informed choices 22, 32, 103
Information 53, 72–3, 103
Institutional model 79
Interactionist approach 14, 34–5,
79–80
symbolic 50

Jay Report 78
Johnson's model 85–6
Joint appointees 108

Knowledge-base 130
changes in 47
development of 32–4, 60
specialist 69

Laissez-faire approach 32
Language 23, 25–6
inappropriate 97
and jargon 11, 41
of nursing model 41
of nursing process 123–4
Leadership 5–6
of clinical team 106
Learning 104
difficulties 81
needs 48
package 72
transfer of 72
Life processes model 81, 84
Linear processes 4
Local authority care 78

McFarlane's charter for nursing 116
Macmillan services 73–5
Management style/system 6, 21, 105,
108
Marie Curie service 75
Maslow 60–1
hierarchy of human needs 62, 84,
92–3
Measuring tools 32, 42–3
Media debate 22
Medical model 10–11, 13, 19, 23, 32,
34, 60
of health care 103
and mental handicap nursing 78–9
and nurse training 120–1, 124
and paediatric nursing 90
and patient education 48
Medical profession 5, 10, 13, 65

Ward records   95
Ward report 105
  in student assessment   123–4
Ward sister   4, 6, 23, 96, 106–7
  and change of role   110–12
  and Salmon Report   108

and teaching of nursing practice
  106
World Health Organisation   81

Zaadie doll   97, 98